LOVE AND MIDWIFERY

This unique book argues that love underpins safe, effective, and high-quality midwifery care, and enables readers to explore sustainable and compassionate ways to engage with their profession.

At a time when midwives are struggling to stay connected with the passion that brought them into the profession, and fear, distress, and trauma are prevalent within maternity care for both staff and those receiving care, this book maps a new way forward. It encourages reflection and discussion about how love impacts midwives' experience of their practice and improves the quality of care they are able to provide for women and their families. It develops a theoretical basis for understanding why love is relevant to midwifery, how midwives think of love, and the ways that it is communicated in practice. It offers practical ways in which love can be appropriately nurtured and applied in contemporary maternity settings, whilst upholding the professional standards required of all maternity care providers. Many chapters include the authentic words of midwives reflecting on the role of love in their own practice experiences.

Love and Midwifery is a valuable contribution to the literature around compassion, kindness, resilience, moral distress, and trauma in maternity care, helping midwives to realise and feel proud of the love in their work. It is an essential read for all midwives from student to experienced practitioner, as well as the wider maternity care workforce.

Diane Ménage is a midwife with a life-long interest in women's health and well-being. Throughout her career, her focus has always been on providing individualised evidence-based care through relationships. As a midwife, she has worked clinically in hospital settings, community midwifery, and independent practice. Diane's PhD explored women's experiences of compassionate midwifery care.

Jenny Patterson has worked as a midwife since 2007, within the UK NHS and independently. Jenny has a particular interest in traumatic birth experiences and her PhD thesis explored post-traumatic stress disorder in women post childbirth (PTSD-PC). Jenny has been part of an international group of midwives, midwifery researchers, and lecturers that explored midwives' needs regarding stress and trauma across the United Kingdom and Ireland.

LOVE AND MIDWIFERY

Edited by Diane Ménage and Jenny Patterson

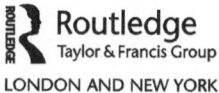

Routledge
Taylor & Francis Group

LONDON AND NEW YORK

Designed cover image: Pixabay, adapted by Lee Patterson

First published 2025
by Routledge
4 Park Square, Milton Park, Abingdon, Oxon OX14 4RN

and by Routledge
605 Third Avenue, New York, NY 10158

Routledge is an imprint of the Taylor & Francis Group, an informa business

British Library Cataloguing-in-Publication Data
A catalogue record for this book is available from the British Library

ISBN: 978-1-032-64576-6 (hbk)
ISBN: 978-1-032-64571-1 (pbk)
ISBN: 978-1-032-64578-0 (ebk)

DOI: 10.4324/9781032645780

Typeset in Times New Roman
by SPi Technologies India Pvt Ltd (Straive)

We dedicate this book to Nicolette Peel M.B.E.
(1972–2023).

CONTENTS

STATEMENT FROM THE EDITORS REGARDING THEIR DECISION ABOUT THE USE OF GENDER INCLUSIVE LANGUAGE IN THIS BOOK

It is important to us as editors that everyone who reads this book feels acknowledged, respected, and included. We have spent considerable time reflecting on how best to present gender-inclusive language. Having read widely, and attended workshops and debates, we see that views, opinions, and understandings are diverse and at times controversial. It is clear that whichever format of language we choose, it might not be acceptable to everyone. This is reflected by McGlothen-Bell et al. (2023), who in their comprehensive examination of gender-inclusive care and women's health do not attempt to specify an appropriate form of language. We agree with their emphasis on the need to review terminology related to gender-nonconforming populations and their known healthcare needs and ensure the provision of gender-equitable and respectful care. We strongly desire to take a loving approach that encompasses individualised, respectful care for every person using maternity services. We call on every reader of this book to reflect on and consider their own approach when they engage with anyone seeking maternity care.

Yet, we needed to decide about the language we would use in this book. We agreed that we would use the term woman in the *sexed* context of female human biology. Thus, we have drawn on the position statement provided by the UK Network of Professors of Midwifery and Maternal and Newborn Health, May (2023), regarding the use of sexed language. Thus:

We use the words women and woman throughout this book, recognising that this reflects the biology and identity of the great majority of those who are childbearing; for the purpose of this book, these terms include girls, and people whose gender identity does not correspond with their birth sex or who may have a non-binary identity. All those using maternal and reproductive healthcare and services should receive individualised, respectful care including use of the gender nouns and pronouns they prefer.

Nevertheless, we fully acknowledged and respected the right of individual authors to have a different approach. Therefore, authors who were not comfortable with the approach described above have used the language they preferred.

References

McGlothen-Bell, K., Greene, M. Z., Hunt, G., & Crawford, A. D. (2023). Intersectional Examination of Gender-Inclusive Care and Women's Health. *Journal of obstetric, gynecologic, and neonatal nursing: JOGNN*, 52(6), 442–453. https://doi.org/10.1016/j. jogn.2023.08.007

UK Network of Professors of Midwifery and Maternal and Newborn Health. (2023). *Position Statement: Use of sexed language in relation to women's reproductive health.* https://www.councilofdeans.org.uk/wp-content/uploads/2024/02/Position-Statement-Use-of-sexed-language-FINAL-May-2023.pdf

ABOUT THE EDITORS

Diane Ménage is a midwife with a life-long interest in women's health and well-being. Throughout her career, her focus has always been on providing individualised evidence-based care through relationships. As a midwife, she has worked clinically in hospital settings, community midwifery, and independent practice. She completed her PhD research on *Women's Lived Experience of Compassionate Midwifery* at Coventry University (UK) in 2018. She has written extensively for midwifery journals, contributed to book chapters and she co-authored the textbook *An Introduction to Research for Midwives, 4th Edition*. Diane is a part-time lecturer in Midwifery at De Montfort University. In her role as a midwifery educator, she is passionate about embedding compassion and self-compassion into midwifery education.

Jenny Patterson has worked as a midwife since 2007, within the UK NHS and independently. Jenny has a particular interest in traumatic birth experiences and Jenny's PhD thesis explored post-traumatic stress disorder in women post childbirth (PTSD-PC). Jenny has been part of an international group of midwives, midwifery researchers, and lecturers that explored midwives' needs regarding stress and trauma across the UK and Ireland. Following completion of trauma management training, Jenny has led workshops for women and midwives. Jenny has published several midwifery journal articles, contributed to a few book chapters and presented in the UK and Europe. Jenny currently lectures in midwifery at Edinburgh Napier University, Scotland, UK. Current research interests include exploring how maternity care providers and interpreters can best collaborate to provide high quality care for women whose first language is not that of the country in which they are receiving maternity care.

CONTRIBUTORS

Anna Byrom Commencing her midwifery career over 24 years ago, Anna has worked in a variety of roles across midwifery services, education, and research, throughout the UK. With a passion for relational, humanised, and rights-based midwifery care for all, she has worked across the UK as a caseload, team and birth centre midwife, and leading infant-feeding services in community and hospital settings. Anna completed her PhD, in 2019, with the Maternal and Infant Nutrition and Nurture Unit (MAINN) at the University of Central Lancashire, England. Her thesis explored the influences of the UNICEF UK Baby Friendly Initiative upon midwives and service-users. Passionate about supporting authentic, relational, and social midwifery education, she was awarded a National Teaching Fellowship, in 2019, from Advance HE, acknowledging her extensive contributions to midwifery education since 2010. Anna is the publisher of The Practising Midwife, Australia Edition and The Student Midwife journals and founding Director/CEO of the award-winning All4Maternity.com supporting the learning, sharing, and caring needs for all midwives and maternity workers. Anna has worked with global, national, regional, and local teams to support internationally educated midwives with their transition to practice across NHS England and has been principal investigator on a number of midwifery education and clinical practice research projects, including Sustaining Midwifery Continuity of Carer in Practice; Collaborative Learning in Practice; and Student Midwife Continuity of Carer placement learning.

Sheena Byrom is a practising midwife of 40 years, having worked in the NHS for most of that time. Sheena was one of the UK's first consultant midwives, and as head of midwifery successfully helped to lead the development of three birth centres in East Lancashire. As well as being an international speaker,

Sheena provides workshops and consultancy services on respectful maternity care, and the support of physiological childbirth. Sheena was awarded an OBE in 2011 for services to midwifery and was made an honorary fellow of the Royal College of Midwives in 2015. In 2016 and 2018, Sheena received honorary doctorates from Bournemouth University and the University of Central Lancashire, and in 2017 she was made a visiting fellow at Bournemouth University. Sheena is committed to the humanisation of childbirth, and to supporting the wellbeing of maternity staff through compassionate, collaborative, and inclusive leadership.

Kate Greenstock is a practising midwife, coach, and facilitator. As a midwife, she worked until recently within an NHS continuity of carer team; as a coach, she supports midwives and others in healthcare to creatively re-imagine their work lives. Her favourite part of being a midwife is witnessing and supporting "newborn" families in their profound transition and changing identities. She brings an absolute conviction that there is no substitute in the world for you, and your unique voice. Kate is a Certified Co-Active Coach (CPCC) and Professional Certified Coach (PCC) with the International Coach Federation (ICF). Kate is a skilled facilitator of groups, shaping leadership development environments for pioneering healthcare professionals, and enjoys creating reflective spaces with midwives and student midwives. She facilitates Schwartz Rounds (exploring the emotional impact of healthcare work) for her home NHS trust. She published her book *Flourish: A Practical and Emotional Guidebook to Thriving in Midwifery* in 2023.

Indie Luna is a classically trained medical anthropologist and clinically trained midwife with a passion for global maternal and neonatal health, and over a decade's international experience in a range of governmental and non-governmental organisations. She is currently the managing director of Atsede Clinic, Ethiopia, whilst also working towards completing a PhD at the London School of Hygiene and Tropical Medicine. Indie has published widely in leading midwifery journals, spoken at international maternal health conferences, participated in GRCF-funded qualitative research projects, and co-authored the book *With Two Souls* (published in 2022) with Gurage midwife Atsede Kidane, reflecting on the unique experiences of birth, death, love, and life in rural Ethiopia. Her second book, *The Midwife's Apprentice*, is due to be published in 2025.

Anna Marsh Since qualifying in 2017, Anna has worked in a busy central London hospital across all areas of maternity care. After completing a Wellbeing of Women Entry Level Scholarship for Midwives, she undertook a NIHR Predoctoral Clinical Academic Fellowship. Her research area of interest is improving how we communicate with women and pregnant people, with particular focus on the use of social media. Anna's current role is in Perinatal Quality Improvement.

Elizabeth Newnham is associate professor of midwifery at Flinders University in Australia. For 25 years, her clinical practice, teaching and research has focused on seeking social justice solutions for humanising birth, currently through the development of four research streams: ethics, technology, environment, and practice. Related work includes critical analysis of birth discourse and policy, exploring the role of bioethics in obstetric violence, and developing care ethics concepts for relational midwifery practice. She has published widely in these areas and been an invited speaker at conferences and events in Europe, the United States, the UK and Australia.

Claire Nutt is a midwifery academic at the University of Birmingham, supporting their BSc midwifery apprenticeships and MSc midwifery programmes for nurses becoming midwives. She previously taught at the University of the West of England. Her midwifery career has included community midwifery, care in a birth centre, as a specialist midwife for perinatal mental health, and professional midwifery advocate. As a massage therapist, Claire's passion for massage throughout the perinatal period has precluded and weaved throughout her midwifery career. Alongside private massage clinics and massage for midwives, Claire continues to teach maternity care professionals massage skills for pregnancy and birth with a focus on partner support.

Maeve O'Connell is an assistant professor of midwifery at Fatima College of Health Sciences (FCHS) in Abu Dhabi, where she co-leads the development and teaching of a CAA accredited bachelor midwifery degree program in the UAE. She has been in this role since 2021, after working as a registered midwife and nurse for 20 years with experience working in Ireland, Bahrain and the UK. She holds a PhD in medicine and health from University College Cork and a master's in advanced practice from King's College London. She is also a Fellow of the Faculty of Nursing and Midwifery at RCSI, Ireland. Maeve's research interests include intrapartum care, fear of childbirth (tokophobia), and perinatal mental health. She has published multiple articles, book chapters, and a Cochrane review on these topics, and has presented her findings at international conferences. She is an associate editor for Women and Birth journal and a peer reviewer for many journals. She is passionate about promoting midwifery and maternal and newborn health and has a strong presence on social media as a nurse and midwife. She aims to advance the evidence-based practice, leadership, and education of midwifery in the UAE and beyond.

Naomi O'Donovan is a registered midwife from Ireland. She has been sharing her love of midwifery with students since 2015 and began teaching full time in University College Cork in 2023. Her advocacy work led her to represent Ireland at the European Midwives Association and International Confederation of Midwives. Naomi has worked throughout Cork University Maternity Hospital and their domino team. Maintaining a clinic in West Cork, she is widely known for her passion for facilitating physiological birth.

Lesley Page Building on a long and intense career in midwifery, Professor Lesley Page CBE works to humanise childbirth, supporting pregnancy, birth, and the early weeks of life as a transformative event that is critical to our future. Lesley served as president of the Royal College of Midwives, UK from April 2012 till June 2017. Lesley has considerable international experience and has worked in, and lectured in, many parts of the world. Lesley became the first professor of midwifery in the UK at Thames Valley University and Queen Charlotte's and Hammersmith Hospitals NHS Trust, London, UK in 2001. She is visiting professor of midwifery in the Florence Nightingale Faculty of Nursing and Midwifery and Palliative Care, King's College London, and adjunct professor at the University of Technology Sydney. Lesley received the International Alumni Award from the University of Technology Sydney in 2013 and was conferred with an honorary DSc by the University of West London in November 2013. In 2014, she was made a Commander of the British Empire (CBE) for services to midwifery. In 2021, Lesley received an honorary PhD in Midwifery from the University of Iceland.

Clare Wardhaugh's original qualification in physical education led her to work as a teacher with adults who had severe to mild learning disabilities. After working in that field for 12 years she then joined a religious community, where she studied for a master's degree in pastoral studies and then person-centred counselling. During this time, she was involved in personal development work in post-communist Lithuania and Croatia following the Balkans war. Also, during these years she developed a holistic approach to counselling and spiritual direction using movement. She was one of the founders of a holistic spirituality centre in Perth, Scotland. After 19 years in religious life, Clare went on to work for 15 years in education teaching religious education with young people aged 12–18 years. Clare now takes time to write and reflect on her life in social work, religious life, counselling, spiritual direction, and in education. In this reflection, she recognises that her life has been a continuing journey of learning what it means to love and to love well. She has listened and learned from all those who have worked with her and accompanied her in her life, she attempts to live in the spirit of gratitude for all that has been and given to her.

Michelle Waterfall has been a registered midwife in England for over 20 years. During her career, she has worked in all areas of maternity in a clinical capacity and gained significant leadership and managerial experience. This lived leadership experience was enhanced when Michelle successfully completed an MBA in 2021. Michelle joined the Northwest Regional Maternity Team in March 2021 and was appointed as the Deputy Regional Chief Midwife in July 2021. She is determined to use this opportunity to support local maternity and neonatal care providers and systems to strive towards high-quality, personalised maternity care.

FOREWORD

To paraphrase the extraordinary late Tina Turner – midwifery, *"what has love got to do with it?,"* I ask this as midwifery, despite being one of the oldest health professions in the world, has been subsumed by technocratic task-based clinical activities, stripping the humanity from "caregiving." The word "care" means to show concern for, kindness to, or empathy for others, but maternity staff frequently work in unrelenting and sometimes, hostile environments reducing their capacity to "care." While "being caring" is relegated to the so-called "soft" skills, with escalating rates of birth trauma and obstetric violence, we know the opposite is true. To feel deeply, to care, to empathise, to provide compassionate care, to emotionally attune and align with another, is to put simply, *extremely* hard. While working this way *is* hard, it also bestows a delightful reciprocal gift that nourishes and restores the giver, fosters a sense of contribution and meaning, allowing staff to move into the next interaction recharged, not depleted. However, the nature of institutionalised and technocratic birth frequently undermines these precious interactions, so much so it may seem outrageous to even consider the concept of love in relation to midwifery care. At first glance, it may feel like we are asking even more of overstretched, under resourced staff. But I posit, that it may just be the antidote that we are looking for...

So, what has love got to do with midwifery care? Well, this book will tell you in exquisite detail and depth. As the first of its kind, with 13 diverse and rich chapters from esteemed authors, the book journeys through different conceptualisations of love as applied to midwifery care. Through this journey, we see love explored in the broadest sense and learn that it is made up of many constituent parts. Crucially, love-as-action is explored extensively through the myriad ways love is expressed in midwifery care, leadership, and education – love as touch, actions, words, time, and a gift to name a few. When reframing these everyday midwifery acts, we come to see love is threaded through all that we do, and this book also offers a clear articulation of the invisible work that midwives do. Centring the emotionality of midwifery interactions, as this book does so beautifully, also offers a book of resistance. Resisting the status quo that accepts birth trauma, obstetric violence, racism (to name a few), or even the tragic state of indifference, this book gently and lovingly challenges us to keep trying to make a difference. Through acknowledging, articulating, and centring love as a crucial component of midwifery, this book is a powerful companion as we go about our work of correcting the course of maternity care.

Dr Claire Feeley
Lecturer and Midwifery/Maternal Health Researcher
King's College London

PREFACE

When we (Diane and Jenny) met in 2017 at a research methods conference, we discovered we had many things in common. Within our personal lives, we shared a passion for growing vegetables and living/travelling in small spaces (Diane on a boat, and Jenny in a campervan). Within our professional lives as midwives, we had both worked within the UK NHS; spent some years in independent practice; trained as supervisors of midwives; and were now both in the midst of PhD research using the same analysis methodology. But of most interest was that each of us in our research was exploring aspects of the way midwives and women experience their interaction or relationships with one another. We determined to keep in touch. We soon realised that although our PhD questions addressed two extremes of the nature of interaction (Diane compassionate experiences, Jenny traumatic experiences), there were underlying parallels in our findings. We completed our PhDs and read each other's PhD theses and were excited at these parallels, which can most appropriately be described collectively as the need to recognise and acknowledge the human beings within, and the humanity of, midwifery. The following quotes depict this core sense of humanity.

"I dunno, there is something wrong in a system that doesn't allow you to feel like a human being" Julie (woman participant) (Patterson et al., 2019, p. 27).

"I think it was her positivity and practical support but she did it in a very compassionate way, a very warm, human way, she was just a person, you know, I didn't get a sense of the uniform if you like." Mary (woman participant) (Menage et al., 2020).

"Humanity is important in any culture and within the NHS it feels like humanity should be core" (West, 2013).

Clearly women need to be seen as individual human beings, but they also take comfort in connecting with the human being in the midwife or other healthcare professional, as both Julie's and Mary's words above illustrate. Moreover, recognition is needed, at organisational level, that midwives themselves are both professional *and* human, in order to support them to care compassionately (Menage et al., 2018).

For a few years, we were delighted and honoured to be given the opportunity to present our research findings together at several UK-wide conferences, as well as to publish a couple of joint articles. As we journeyed through this time, we were both being drawn to a word that had been briefly raised in our theses, but which was not easily raised in midwifery circles:

Love

As practising midwives, then midwifery researchers, and now midwifery lecturers, we have experienced and witnessed first-hand the compassion as well as the distress and trauma that exists within the maternity care environment both for staff and those receiving care. The antidote to fear and distress, we and many others believe, is love. The need for love within our human interactions is beautifully summed up by the Dalai Lama:

> *"Some people consider the practice of love and compassion is only related to religious practice and if they are not interested in religion, they neglect these inner values. But love and compassion are qualities that human beings require just to live together."*
>
> *(Dalai Lama, n.d.)*

Then in August 2022, during an online meeting between us, Diane said "Jenny I've a growing idea I want to put to you…I'd like us to write a book". Jenny replied "Oh yes, up for that…what about?." "Love" said Diane, "Yes, absolutely" was the reply without hesitation. And so, this book was conceived.

From the outset, it was clear that this book had a life of its own. We were midwives overseeing, perhaps facilitating, the gestation and birth of a book that we felt was vital for our time. We had some important questions to answer and decisions to make. We very quickly realised we didn't have the expertise between us to write the whole book and that it would be richer and more valuable if we invited other authors to contribute. The question then was how to choose from the very many renowned midwifery authors and the many midwives and others we both knew who had much to offer for this book. We had many conversations. We followed up suggestions and connections and through a fairly organic process the collective of authors became clear. Yet, we are very aware of many others who would have also had much to contribute, and we acknowledge you and say, perhaps there will be a second book.

Indeed, this book is merely a drop in the ocean of all that could be written and explored around love and midwifery, but we believe it counts.

References

Dalai Lama. (n.d.). AZQuotes.com. Retrieved October 30, 2024, from AZQuotes.com. https://www.azquotes.com/quote/811702

Menage, D., Bailey, E., Lees, S., & Coad, J. (2018). *Women's Lived Experience of Compassionate Midwifery. Doctoral Thesis.* Coventry University. https://www.researchgate.net/publication/385449575_Women's_Lived_Experience_of_Compassionate_Midwifery

Menage, D., Bailey, E., Lees, S., & Coad, J. (2020). Women's lived experience of compassionate midwifery: Human and professional. *Midwifery, 85,* 102662. https://doi.org/10.1016/j.midw.2020.102662

Patterson, J., Hollins Martin, C. J., & Karatzias, T. (2019). Disempowered midwives and traumatised women: Exploring the parallel processes of care provider interaction that contribute to women developing Post Traumatic Stress Disorder (PTSD) post childbirth. *Midwifery, 76,* 21–35. https://doi.org/10.1016/j.midw.2019.05.010

West, M. (2013, March 7). *Developing cultures of high-quality care.* https://www.kingsfund.org.uk/insight-and-analysis/videos/michael-west-developing-cultures-high-quality-care#:~:text=That%20staff%20views%20of%20their,to%20staff%20satisfaction%20as%20well

ACKNOWLEDGEMENTS

There are so many people who we wish to acknowledge for their inspiration, support, and guidance as we brought this book together. We would particularly like to thank Clare Cable, who planned to co-write a chapter, but due to family bereavement needed to step down. Nevertheless, Clare contributed much to our thinking and development of content through valuable conversations at the start of this journey. Thanks to Ann Oakley for her positive confirmation of the value in the book as well as access to her article.

We would also like to thank those we spoke to who were at first hesitant about the nature of this book. These conversations added balance and ensured our careful reflection on the structure and content of the book. We especially wish to acknowledge Catherine Williams whose initial reflection on this topic gave us lots of food for thought.

Other midwives….

We thank the many midwives who were happy to have a chance to talk about the love in their work and who shared their personal thoughts, feelings, and experiences. It was when we talked to midwives about the love in their work that we noticed just how much this meant to them. There was a sense of relief and excitement, yet many were moved to tears. They told us that they had never had the chance to talk about this before and it was listening to midwives and student midwives talk about love that showed how important it was to bring this book into being. Although it was only possible to present a small fraction of their words within specific chapters of this book, everything they told us has contributed in some way. Special thanks to Jane Dobson for her support and enthusiasm for discussing all things related to midwifery and love over a curry.

We are hugely indebted to each of the wonderful authors who have contributed to the book. Their vision, expertise, and dedication shine through and have made this book what it is. We certainly could not have done it without them.

Our thanks to Routledge who very quickly affirmed our proposal for this book and confirmed their backing for the production and provided sustained support throughout. We are grateful to Claire Feeley for very generously taking the time to read our manuscript and write a beautiful foreword.

Finally, our gratitude to our husbands Lee and Jem, who have stood by us throughout this journey and offered not only love and support, but hands on practical support with proof-reading and reflection (Jem) and wonderful image design and production especially for our front cover and conclusion (Lee).

INTRODUCTION

Introduction

The journey began with a literature search for any writing about love *and* midwifery, and to be honest, it was a bit desert-like, with imagined proverbial tumbleweed. We found very little literature directly speaking about love. Literature about compassion and relationships, yes, but love? A similar search regarding love *and* nursing returned a greater number of articles; we discovered that the idea of love, as a feature of professional practice, has been explored a little more in nursing. A key nursing care theorist, Jean Watson, views love as a transformative force in nursing suggesting that "Rather than asking: *how can we dare to bring love and caring together into our lives and work? We can ask: how can we bear not to?*" (Watson, 2003, p. 200). Marlienne Goldin (2019) found that even though love is not a term heard often in healthcare, loving care is central to nursing, with "love of humanity manifested in nursing practice" (p. 318). Also, there is a recent valuable concept analysis exploring love in nursing (Adib-Hajbaghery & BolandianBafghi, 2020). In medicine, several doctors have considered love in their practice, including palliative care doctor and author Dr Rachel Clarke, whose book *Dear Life: A Doctor's Story of Love and Loss* explored the profound impact of love and human connection in the face of death in her work at a hospice (Clarke, 2020). We dug a little deeper and were able to find some more literature on the topic of love and midwifery, but still not much. This strongly cemented our decision that this book needed to be brought to life. Next, we provide a brief overview of some of the papers and sources we discovered in considering the value of this book.

DOI: 10.4324/9781032645780-1

The earliest article we found that directly referred to midwifery and love was the William Power Memorial lecture by the sociologist Ann Oakley in 1989 entitled "Who cares for women? Science versus love in midwifery today" (Oakley, 1989). We were unable to source a copy and so wrote to Ann and she very kindly sent us one. Ann carefully explores the history of the oft experienced divide between medical and midwifery approaches to childbirth, while emphasising that to remain within a language of opposition is misleading and hinders progress towards collaboration that can optimise childbearing experience and outcomes. Science versus love? Here science relates to growth in technology and medical interventions and love relates to caring and social approaches. Ann Oakley (1989) assesses the evidence on the safety and effectiveness of caring, "What the scientific value of love is, if you like?" (p. 217), she concludes that "love is a scientific concept and its effects on perinatal health can be quantified" (p. 219). Ann's summary that "love – caring – is as important as science...in maternity services" (p. 219) is explored in Chapter 8 that discusses the concepts of *Vigil of Care* and *Care as Gift*. Interestingly, another early source was a report from the 22nd International Congress for Midwifery in Kobe, Japan, in 1990. The article was in Swedish, the title was "Love, skill and knowledge – a midwife's gifts" (Persson et al., 1991). In 1999, Michel Odent published his seminal work *The scientification of love* (Odent, 1999). He argued that love mattered in midwifery work in society at that time. He tells us that our experience of birth (as newborns) is critical to the development of the ability to love and that the survival of humankind, in the face of climate and political crises, relies more than ever on cooperation and love rather than violence. The work by Kerstin Uvnäs-Moberg (2011) on oxytocin, often referred to as the hormone of love, provides a strong physiological basis for the role of love. Sue Barker in her book presenting her research of midwives' emotional care of women draws on work by both nursing and midwifery theorists to provide a strong focus on love as a component in midwifery, suggesting that care, as a form of *moderated love* or *loving relationship*, is unique to midwifery (Barker, 2011, p. 47). A few years later, the work by Sue Gerhardt (2015) sets out the role of love in childhood development; while not specifically midwifery-focussed, it adds to the understanding of love in the context of childbearing.

Nicolette Peel (2016), midwife and founding member of the Mummy's Star charity, did not shy away from using the word love. In an article she wrote in 2016, she highlighted that within midwifery a very particular magic of our craft is to relate and communicate. Peel called on us to remember that each woman, midwife, colleague, and manager has a warm, vulnerable, human-beating heart. When we acknowledge this humanity, we are more able to understand, unite, and love. Nicolette concluded:

I believe that courage is the way forward, kindness is the healer and love is the answer.

(Peel, 2016, p. 9)

Television series often reflect human experience. Stephen McGann, best known as the actor who plays the part of Dr Turner in the popular TV series *Call the Midwife*, based on the memoirs of East London midwife Jennifer Worth in the 1950s and 1960s, was invited to speak at the UK Royal College of Midwives annual conference in 2017. McGann, an actor not a doctor, said he was amazed at the popularity of the series and had met and spoken to many midwives and doctors over the previous few years. He was particularly interested in why the series was so popular. Those he spoke to invariably put it down, not to historical or even clinical accuracy, but because it was about love (McGann, 2017).

Finally, during the process of creating this book, we were directed to a book by Spanish midwife Consuelo Ruiz Velez-Frias entitled *Midwives: an ancestral profession based on love*, an historic account of the evolution and erasure of midwifery in Spain in the 20th century (Velez-Frias, 1998). While in Spanish and now unavailable, Maria Velo Higueras, a midwifery lecturer at Robert Gordon University, has a copy and told us that "The book comes from the love of Consuelo, who was making a last plea, in her last days, for her beautiful profession not to disappear...as midwives were almost entirely replaced by obstetric nurses." In the book, Consuelo reflected on how "the love for the profession was the only thing that could bring it back" (Velo Higueras, 2024).

So now we felt, as Jean Watson said, "We have a new call to bring us back to that which resides deep within us...the latent love within our caring work" (Watson, 2003, p. 198).

With this in mind, we began to discuss our plan for this book with many people and potential authors. Around this time, we put out a call on Twitter "Does love have a role in midwifery?" The overall response was clear: *yes, of course there is love in midwifery*. The post below is just one example.

> I say YES YES YES. We should talk about it more. All the relationships we work with are centred around connection and emotions, which to me is love!
> In response to post on X (formerly Twitter) by Claire (midwife)

Yet, there were a few hesitations. *Is it professional to speak of love? What sort of love?* These hesitations highlighted something we were both aware of; within healthcare, words such as compassion, empathy, kindness, and respect are deemed acceptable, but *love* is a rarely used yet powerful four-letter word. Others have written of this hesitancy and that perhaps in response to fear or ridicule we choose not to refer to *love* but rather *positive regard* and maintaining *professional distance* (Mahon, 2016). One person sent us a reflection on why they had a visceral reaction to the idea of love and midwifery. Concerns included the appropriate use of boundaries and the complexity of power differentials with potential for abuse of power, both with women and colleagues.

Taking the range of responses into account, we both, like Eva Luckes, a contemporary of Florence Nightingale and matron of the Royal London

Hospital (Mahon, 2016), had a strongly held belief in the rightness of referring to love *and* midwifery.

The structure of the book

This book is an exploration of what we mean by love in the context of maternity care. It is also a celebration of the myriad experiences of love shared with us during the process of writing and editing this book, by midwives, student midwives, obstetricians, and many more whose lives are intertwined with birth and midwifery. Some of these people's words are presented in this book with permission, using their name if they wanted this, or otherwise using a pseudonym or just "anonymous."

Part I: *Love in Context* explores and discusses various theories and perspectives on love. The aim is to address the uneasiness that can arise when speaking of love in the context of midwifery by providing a strong basis and understanding of what we mean by love and, importantly, why it matters in midwifery. In Chapter 1, the nature of love and different ways to understand love are discussed from perspectives such as theology, philosophy, and physiology. The beautiful letters of Chapter 2 set the ground for the place of love in midwifery, particularly the humanity of midwifery. Chapter 3 serves to provide a strong theoretical basis and rationale for why we believe we need to talk about love in midwifery. It draws on care ethics to position love as a solution to maternity care crises such as violence, abuse, and dehumanisation – a solution that builds towards humanised ethical practice through human connection.

From this strong basis, Part II: *Love in Practice* explores possible pathways of practice structured around the five languages of love as proposed by Gary Chapman (2015). Although Chapman's focus is on relationships with partners, which is not what this book is about, we believe each of these five languages is very relevant within midwifery practice: touch, acts, words, time, and gift.

Being mindful of the professional nature of midwifery, Part III: *Love in the Profession* widens the discussion to explore the role of love within the midwifery profession. First, Chapter 9 explores how love can be understood within the context of midwives taking care of themselves and thus sustainability. Chapter 10 looks at the role of love within the midwifery workplace in terms of colleagues and workplace culture. Chapters 11 and 12 go on to explore the place of love with midwifery leadership and midwifery education. Chapter 13 brings together a discussion of love in the context of the professional role and considers four specific areas: relational care, professional boundaries, the contribution of research, and culture change.

The aim of this book is to help midwives realise and feel proud of the love in their work. We want this book to secure a (long overdue) place for love in discussions about midwifery care. We see it as kick-starting the conversation and acting as a catalyst for further exploration and collaboration on this topic in the years to come.

We hope that as you journey through this book, or indeed as you dip into the sections that you feel drawn to, you will gain a sense of the understanding, even conviction, that love should start to be spoken about more in midwifery.

You may have wondered why there is a diamond on the cover of this book. Read on and gradually the reason will reveal itself.

References

Adib-Hajbaghery, M., & BolandianBafghi, S. (2020). Love in nursing: a concept analysis. *Journal of caring sciences, 9*(2), 113–119. https://doi.org/10.34172/JCS.2020.017

Barker, S. (2011). *Midwives' emotional care of women becoming mothers.* Cambridge Scholars Publishing.

Chapman, G. (2015). *The five love languages: the secret to love that lasts.* Moody.

Clarke, R. (2020). *Dear Life: A doctor's story of love, loss and consolation.* Little Brown.

Gerhardt, S. (2015). *Why love matters: How affection shapes a baby's brain* (2nd ed). Routledge.

Goldin, M. (2019). Nursing as love: A hermeneutical phenomenological study of creative thought within nursing. *International Journal for Human Caring, 23*(4), 312–319. https://doi.org/10.20467/1091-5710.23.4.312

Mahon, S. (2016). Love matters. *The Practising Midwife, 19*(3), 42.

McGann, S. (2017). *Royal College of Midwives conference presentation.* Manchester.

Oakley, A. (1989). William Power Memorial Lecture. Who cares for women? Science versus love in midwifery today. *Midwives Chronicle,* 214–221.

Odent, M. (1999). *The scientification of love.* Free Association Books.

Peel, N. (2016). Love is a cold climate: Midwifery and politics. *Midwifery Matters, 150,* 8–9.

Persson, E., Wahlbom, A., & Gottvall, K. (1991). Rapporter från den 22:a Internationella kongressen för barnmorskor i Kobe, Japan, mellan den 7-12 okt 1990. "A midwife's gift--love, skill and knowledge" [Report from the 22d International Congress for Midwives in Kobe, Japan between 7 and 12 Oct. 1990. "A midwife's gift--love, skill and knowledge"]. *Jordemodern, 104*(1–2), 18–26.

Uvnäs-Moberg, K. (2011). *The oxytocin factor: Tapping the hormone of calm, love and healing.* Pinter & Martin Ltd.

Velo Higueras, M. (2024). Personal communication. Twitter.

Velez-Frias, C.R. (1998). *Midwives: An ancestral profession based on love.* Spanish Midwifery Association.

Watson, J. (2003). Love and caring. Ethics of face and hand—An invitation to return to the heart and soul of nursing and our deep humanity. *Nursing Administration Quarterly, 27*(3), 197–202. https://doi.org/10.1097/00006216-200307000-00005

PART I

Love in context

1

WHAT DO WE MEAN BY LOVE?

Diane Ménage

Introduction

The word *love* encapsulates many different ideas, thoughts, emotions and experiences. The love between a mother and baby is clearly different from the love
of a partner or what we feel for a close friend, and these differ again from the
love of a particular piece of music or a place. The idea of being *in-love* is deeply
ingrained in many cultures and emphasised in music, films and literature. So, it
is important to deal with this first. Being *in-love* is sometimes described as a
state of intense wanting and desire (Medaris, 2018), which marks the early days
of a romantic relationship. The wanting and desire may pre-date the actual
relationship and can be there, even when no relationship develops, as in unre-
quited love. Falling in love can be associated with a type of melancholy or
lovesickness which can bring emotional pain and even physical symptoms
(Medaris, 2018). No wonder it has been described as a type of madness. Yet, it
can also be a source of great joy and happiness and a driver for establishing
meaningful relationships. This passionate love is different to compassionate
love, which is associated with more well-established, long-term relationships
(Hatfield, 1989). Indeed, it has been observed that passionate love loses its
intensity, on average, within two years, after which it may (or may not) gradually transition into a long-lasting love. All experiences of love are unique and
complex; therefore, this very brief description of falling in love cannot do justice to all the ways in which people experience love. The idea of being *in-love*
has only been discussed here in order to set it apart, because it is not the focus
of this chapter or this book. That kind of love is important; after all, for many
people, it is the catalyst for finding partners and having babies. But this chapter
will explore the role of different sorts of love, through various lenses and how
love is highly relevant to our lives and work in maternity care.

DOI: 10.4324/9781032645780-3

So, what are the different sorts of love? To answer this, we take a brief trip through some of the many ideas and theories of love, including historical, religious, philosophical and physiological perspectives. This chapter will also explore the relationship between love and concepts such as attachment, compassion and caring to appreciate how difficult it is to pin down and define it and yet how fundamental it is to human life. Along the way, we will also identify how it is inextricably linked to reproduction and human connection.

Historical and religious ideas about love

The ancient Greeks recognised many different forms of love, including *eros*, which is related to passionate, sexual and romantic love; *philia*, which is referred to friendship, affectionate regard and human solidarity (the word philanthropy comes from this); *ludus*, a playful form of love; and *storge*, which is referred to familial and parental love. The highest form of love, according to Aristotle, was *agape* as this was the love from God. However, the meaning of agape has changed and expanded over time and the contemporary meaning of agape can be described as selfless, unconditional love for all beings. These ancient Greek interpretations (particularly agape love) have been developed and integrated into many different religions that see love as a good and powerful quality, and which is central to religious life. For example, in Christianity, The Bible says, "God is love" (*The New Revised Standard Version Bible*, 1995, 1 John 4:8,16) and love for all people was a central feature of Jesus' message. It is manifested in the Muslim religion and the Qur'an has guidance on all sorts of love, including love of God, love for neighbours, family love and friendship (Bin Mohammed, 2019). Love is also very much a part of Judaism; for example, one of the key commandments is to love thy neighbour as thyself (*The Orthodox Jewish Bible*, 2011, Leviticus 19:17-18).

Hinduism states that God is love and that love expresses itself in service (*seva* or sewa as it is known in Hinduism and in Sikhism). Una Viswanathan, a Hindu philanthropist, teacher and thinker, has a special interest in the role of love in Hinduism. She says that

> Love is not just an emotion, it's our very existence, it's woven through all of creation. And the more we see it, the more we experience it, it allows our life to become an expression of that love.
>
> *(Plummer, 2023)*

Buddhism recognises different kinds of love and each of these has something to say about how we can be loving towards ourselves and others (Sheth, 2006). These include:

- Loving-kindness (maitri): being kind to all, caring and nurturing.
- Compassion (karuna): the recognition of suffering in another (or self) and the motivation and the willingness to try to reduce it.

- Appreciative joy (mudita): valuing the now, acknowledging the fleeting nature of life and appreciating everything in it.
- Equanimity (upeksha): mental calmness, seeking to understand rather than react (to others' actions, for example).

These four faces of love tell us that love can make the world a better place and that loving others can help us feel connected and increase our wellbeing. Loving-kindness is a great example of this. The basic premise of loving-kindness is very similar to *the golden rule*: treating others as you wish others to treat you. The golden rule is a universally accepted principal in that some form of it can be found in all religions and schools of thought, from ancient times until the present (Rakhshani, 2017). Loving-kindness is a caring inclusiveness that recognises how connected we all are (Salzberg, 2011). Meditations on loving-kindness have been developed and used by many people and this is discussed further in the section *Love and psychology*.

Love and compassion

Love and compassion are distinct concepts, but they are closely connected, and both involve a concern for the wellbeing of others. Compassion has been defined as "a sensitivity to suffering of self and others, with a commitment to try to alleviate and prevent it" (Gilbert, 2017). Therefore, it arises from a place of empathy and understanding, prompting individuals to act to alleviate suffering and offer support. In maternity care, there is a resistance to talking about suffering and this may be because it is associated with distressing and negative experiences (Byrom et al., In print). However, during the antenatal, intrapartum and postnatal period, women's suffering may not just be discomfort, pain and other physical symptoms. It may also include feeling frightened, overwhelmed, vulnerable, lonely, disempowered, embarrassed, sad, disappointed, frustrated, angry, heartbroken and not good enough, to name just a few of the ways in which women can experience suffering. For those who shrink from the word suffering, perhaps try substituting it for any of these. Compassionate midwives notice women who are struggling with any of the above and they seek ways of alleviating it. Women want compassion from maternity care staff at these times and it can be a powerful intervention. In a UK study, women who were treated with compassion (by midwives) felt less frightened and more able to cope (Menage et al., 2020).

But the question is: what motivates us to be compassionate? One way to look at this is to see love as the force behind compassion. When we love someone, we are naturally inclined to feel compassion towards them if they are suffering. The same can be said when we work lovingly as midwives and maternity workers. Love fosters empathy and a sense of connection, which in turn drives compassion. Conversely, compassion can deepen and strengthen love. When we demonstrate compassion towards others, we not only alleviate their suffering but also nurture our relationships with them. Moreover, love is not just a driver of compassion for individual people, it can motivate individuals and communities to work towards creating a more just and equitable society. For example, Martin Luther King, the civil rights leader, believed that the power of love, understood as a form of compassionate action, could overcome hatred and injustice and bring about social change (King, 1963).

Love, connection and spirituality

In her book *Atlas of the Heart*, Brené Brown (2021) wisely suggests that defining love might be best left to poets, artists and songwriters. However, she, like us, is committed to making sense of the word and to that end has worked with a team of researchers to develop a draft definition and to test it with further data. The emerging definition from her work is as follows:

> We cultivate love when we allow our most vulnerable and powerful selves to be deeply seen and known, and when we honour the spiritual connection that grows from that offering with trust, respect, kindness, and affection.
>
> *(Brown, 2021, p. 187)*

The theme of nurturing and growth is developed by Brown, who goes on to say,

> Love is not something we give or get; it is something that we nurture and grow, a connection that can be cultivated between two people only when it exists within each one of them – we can love others only as much as we love ourselves.
>
> *(Brown, 2021, p. 185)*

This presents a significant challenge to all of us. There are days when our self-esteem is low, and self-love feels absent. For many, this is further complicated by trauma. A systematic review found that adverse childhood experiences occurred more often among health and social care workers than in the general population. They were also associated with poorer physical and mental health, and increased workplace stress (Mercer et al., 2023). As we consider the definition of love we should remember that our ability to love ourselves and others can be significantly affected by our childhood experiences and past trauma.

The eminent psychiatrist and writer M. Scott Peck, in his bestselling book *The Road Less Travelled* (2002), defined love as

> The will to extend oneself for the purpose of nurturing one's own or another's spiritual growth.
>
> *(p. 81)*

Both Scott Peck and Brown see spiritual growth and love as closely linked. For many years, nursing and midwifery education taught spirituality as respecting the religious traditions of those we care for. However, as professionals, exploring our own spirituality can feel uncomfortable. Most of us have a sense of our spiritual growth, connecting with the things that feed our soul. This may be through a faith tradition, or other ways such as walking in nature, singing in a choir, a mindfulness practice, tai chi or in the company of those we love. Sometimes we find that place of true flourishing through sharing with others, coaching, counselling or spiritual direction.

The challenge of Scot Peck and Brown's definitions of love is that we are invited to reflect upon our own spiritual growth as a starting point. It is in knowing ourselves and being committed to our own development that we can be truly present in a therapeutic relationship with others. Kate Greenstock describes this beautifully in her book *Flourish* (Greenstock, 2023) and brings some practical suggestions for midwives on how to reconnect with ourselves and our purpose. Despite the various forms of love, it is always about the experience of connection and belonging. It comes from a fundamental human need to feel rooted and *at home* in this world. Feeling psychologically *at home* means we experience comfort from having a sense of identity, belonging and being accepted (May, 2011). Understanding our human need to feel *at home* helps us to understand the difficulties of working in challenging maternity environments (where we may not feel *at home*) and why we sometimes do not love it.

Love and philosophy

There are those who consider love to be impossible to pin down, stating that it is philosophically unknowable. Others see love as something that has many manifestations and can be directed towards a wide variety of people, objects and experiences. This is not just the different types of love that were identified by the Greeks and other civilisations but also because ideas around love have changed (and continue to change) over time. Contemporary philosophers point out that love is highly related to the linguistics, culture, norms and values of society. Love can create joy and contentment, but it can also cause great pain. Some manifestations of love are more stable than others with agape love more stable than eros love, for example (Moseley, 2023).

Philosophy invites us to consider love's relationship with power and the potential for the lover to manipulate and control. Others, like Kant, argue that true love is a mutual and freely chosen commitment between individuals, based on respect, autonomy and the recognition of each other's moral worth (Helm, 2021). These opposing ideas can be understood better by considering the different types of love already described in this chapter and the difference between *immature, self-centred* love and *mature, selfless* love (Fromm, 1956). But do all types of love have anything in common? Some philosophers have noted that the effect of loving another person is that it enables someone to see another's *value* or special worth. Scheler argued that the act of valuing somebody or something is an act from the heart (Scheler, 2023, as cited in Helm, 2021). It is easy to imagine that when we see another person's special worth it will be linked to feeling of care towards them. But does love come first and make us see the other person's specialness and worth, or do we see something special in the person first that leads to loving them and caring about them? This is open to debate, but it is possible that they develop simultaneously, and in fact, some argue that valuing and caring are one and the same thing (Seidman, 2009). This ability to see somebody or even something's *specialness* and unique worth would appear a fundamental aspect of all forms of love whether it is love for a new baby, a dear friend, a family pet and even the profession that you love. If we understand this, we can relate it to midwifery care. We see that new parents recognise the unique specialness in *their* baby who is definitely like no other baby in the world, to them. We also know that as we care for women and their families and get to know them (particularly when there is continuity of carer) we develop a relationship through which individualised, compassionate care can be delivered. In other words, when we do not see them as just another *patient* but we see them as unique, special human beings, we can provide care lovingly.

Love and physiology

At a physiological level, humans experience the emotions of love as a result of neurobiological mechanisms regulated by specific neural pathways in the central nervous system. It is a complex phenomenon involving brain activity, key hormones and neurotransmitters, which are produced in the hypothalamus (including oxytocin and vasopressin), and which promote strong feelings of attachment (Marazziti et al., 2021). Alongside this, dopamine makes love feel pleasurable while serotonin and endorphins influence emotional state and mood. Cortisol levels also seem to be involved, particularly in new love, leading to feelings of excitement and stress (Schwartz & Olds, 2015). This complex interplay of hormones is likely to vary according to the nature of the love and the individual.

In midwifery, we place particular emphasis on the role of oxytocin, which is often referred to as the *love hormone*. We understand that it has a pivotal role in both falling in love and bonding and attachment but that it also has a role in labour and birth. It is oxytocin that stimulates uterine contractions during labour. As contractions increase in frequency and intensity, more oxytocin is produced, creating a positive feedback loop (Walter et al., 2021). If all is well, the woman's oxytocin will be produced and do its work. However, if frightened or distressed, adrenaline can block oxytocin, slowing down or stalling labour (Buckley, 2015). This is one of the reasons why women in labour need to feel safe in an environment that is as relaxing, comfortable and stress-free as possible, accompanied by a person or people they love. Most midwives understand this because they have seen women, who have been labouring well at home, arrive at the maternity unit as planned, only for labour to stop. It is easy to see that women who have not been greeted in a calm and caring way when they arrive and are put into a clinical room containing an array of scary equipment with an instruction to "wait for a midwife to come and assess you" are particularly at risk. The body identifies a possible threat in that it is not sure whether this is a safe place to birth. As a result, fear leads to the release of adrenaline, this blocks oxytocin and labour does not progress well. This is why there is a physiologically sound rationale in creating calm, comfortable, homely birthing environments; these are not achieved just by the lighting, furnishings, etc. (although these can be helpful) but also involve providing midwifery in a *loving* way so that women can build trust and feel truly cared for and safe.

Oxytocin also plays a role in the delivery of the placenta. Interactions between the mother and baby as they meet each other for the first time (involving all the senses), stimulate further oxytocin release and the uterus starts to contract again. This is a vital part of the physiological process of the third stage of labour in which the placenta is expelled, and haemostasis is achieved. What is relevant here is that we consider how the love between a mother and their new baby is not just an emotional thing; it involves the complex interplay between physiological and hormonal processes which have important functions during labour, birth, third stage and beyond. Indeed, studies have found that skin-to-skin contact and breastfeeding immediately after birth increase oxytocin levels (Aydin Kartal et al., 2022), reduce postpartum haemorrhage rates for women (at any level of risk) and can decrease the duration of the third stage and the need for intervention (Karimi et al. 2019; Saxton et al. 2015). For this reason, midwives learn that protecting the time immediately after birth, as a time for mother and baby closeness, skin-to-skin contact and initiation of breastfeeding has huge benefits for mother and baby and is therefore a fundamental part of their care. Moreover, understanding the physiological aspects of love (including the role of oxytocin) around the time of birth reveals that it is a key factor in reproduction and the survival of the species.

The dark side to oxytocin

Although oxytocin is known for its ability to promote infant attachment, it also strengthens many types of social bonding in humans. However, in some people and in some circumstances, oxytocin has been linked to lack of trust, intergroup conflict and prejudice (De Dreu, 2016). While not fully understood, a key factor in this is seeing people as *not one of us*; this is sometimes called *othering* (Mercado, 2023). Oxytocin strengthens in-group relationships but appears to have the opposite effect on out-group relationships. The consequences of othering and holding *us* and *them* attitudes (Lephard, 2024) are discussed further in Chapters 10 and 13 in relation to working relationships.

Love and evolution

Love can be seen as an adaptation which is evident in almost all humans, other mammals and possibly some birds. It has a very important function in reproduction, raising young, building communities and survival of the species. It is important to remember that humans are mammals and generally mammals are not born *ready-to-go* in the way that most fish, reptiles and amphibians are. Species differ a lot in the degree and duration of dependency, but human babies are the most dependent of all. Human babies' brains are comparatively underdeveloped at birth, and this means that they cannot do anything for themselves. They cannot even support their own heads. They are reliant on their mothers, fathers or other primary caregivers for their survival.

In this context, we can see that maternal love for a baby is an evolved response and is entirely necessary for survival (Buss, 2018, p. 42; Longrich, 2020). The bond between mother and baby *is* love and any discussion of birthing that does not treat love as a central issue is missing the point. The mother–child bond depends on this deep and visceral emotion. Who knows how many millions of years ago it started, but it seems obvious that a fundamental reproductive strategy of mammals (whose offspring need to be suckled, protected and educated for a long time before they achieve independence) required the evolution of a strong emotion that would motivate the mother to provide the necessary care. We might say that the mother is *biologically programmed* to love her babies and they are programmed to love their mother back, reinforcing the behaviour that ensures their survival.

The fantastic thing about our species is how this primal love has developed in so many ways to play a part in different types of bonding within and outside of families, in communities and social groups. Arguably, all other loves, including paternal love, romantic love, compassion and altruism, can be seen as culturally evolved emotions built on the biological capacity to love that we possess as mammals. It is as if this first experience of love from the mother or other primary caregiver is the blueprint for all other types of love (Longrich, 2020). Therefore, paying attention to love in midwifery is not just a good idea, it is fundamental because love and birthing are intertwined. Pregnancy, birth and the early days with a new baby are times to nurture and pay attention to love. It is where *mothering* is at the very heart of love.

Love and attachment

Love can be seen as the catalyst for primary attachment or bonding. Bowlby (1997, p. 194) described attachment as "lasting psychological connectedness between human beings." A baby's first attachment is usually with their mother, but it can be their father or when parents are not available, another person providing their care. This primary attachment is firstly about survival, but it appears to have a significant impact on attachments with others throughout life (Young et al., 2019). In midwifery, we are familiar with this, and we understand the importance of attachment and we learn that there are things that we can do to support it such as protecting the time immediately after birth (golden hour), encouraging skin-to-skin contact and rooming-in so that mothers and babies are kept together if at all possible. Midwives also have a role to play in supporting the mother/baby dyad and understanding how this reciprocal relationship is fundamental to a good start in life and beyond. They can provide practical support and information to new parents, for example, information on the benefits of responsive feeding and teaching them how to recognise their baby's feeding cues. Sadly, interventionist approaches such as immediate weighing and bathing of babies after birth, strict feeding schedules and separating newborn babies in a nursery (common in many maternity units in the past and still practised in some parts of the world) can be barriers to the start of a loving and intimate relationship between mother and baby.

Love and psychology

Psychological perspectives on love encompass cognitive, emotional, social and behavioural dimensions. Psychologically, Burunat (2016) suggests love does not appear to be an emotion in itself (although it involves emotions); it appears to be a strong physiological drive or motivation, in the same way we are motivated by hunger, thirst and the need for sleep. This is a useful way of looking at love, because it means that for humans, with very few exceptions, *love is something we have already* and not something that is out there somewhere if only it could be found.

Although love is most often defined as a noun, the more astute theorists of love acknowledge that we would all love better if we used it as a verb (hooks, 2001). It is the act of loving somebody or something that makes us feel good. There is considerable evidence that the practice of loving-kindness meditation, which promotes positive emotions, such as joy, gratitude and connection, has wide-ranging benefits for health and wellbeing (Neff, 2011). Loving-kindness practices promote compassion towards oneself and others, and this can improve wellbeing and strengthen relationships. A systematic review carried out to assess the benefits of loving-kindness meditation for those working in caring professions concluded that it should be considered a strategy to reduce stress, ease empathic distress and increase positive affect (Watson et al., 2023). Loving-kindness can be seen as one of the three elements of *self-compassion*, the other two being self-kindness and mindfulness (Neff, 2011). This aspect of love can be rewarding in our personal lives and professional roles. Indeed, participating in loving-kindness practices has been found to be an effective tool to improve empathy and communication skills and reduce compassion fatigue in doctors and nurses (Chen et al., 2021; Asadollah et al., 2023). Although there is little research into its use with midwives, these studies and others suggest it may have a lot to offer.

Love and doing

Love as a verb is likely to resonate with midwives. Loving is about *being alongside* and it is experienced in our actions. We know when we see an interaction that conveys love; we are hard wired to recognise and experience its presence. It is also dynamic. Love has continual movement as we change and grow both as individuals and professionals. It changes day to day, hour to hour. There are times when we may not feel warmth towards ourselves or another, but as midwives we can *choose* to act lovingly. Choosing to embody love as a verb, M. Scott Peck (2002) sums this up well:

> Love is as love does. Love is an act of will-namely, both an intention and an action. Will also implies choice. We do not have to love. We choose to love.
>
> *(p. 83)*

Scott Peck challenges the popular assumption that we love instinctively, but rather that we can all choose to act with love. Loving is an experience which involves thinking, feeling and doing. Loving can be the most powerful and overwhelming experience, but it does not have to be. It can also be the hundreds of little things you experience. The glimpses of loving may be found in the smile, in the tending of a plant, in the cup of tea that you made somebody. Andrews (2010) came up with 30 words to help us understand love in all its aspects. He calls these the *heartwarmings*, see Box 1.1.

Andrews points out that these words provide us with many ways and opportunities to *be loving* and they all represent a positive response to what or who is loved. What is more, Andrews proposes that this sort of loving is an act of will and something that we can *choose* to build into our lives. The potential to be loving is already within us. It might be helpful to try the activity in Box 1.2.

BOX 1.1 ANDREW'S HEARTWARMINGS

Affection, alertness, appreciation, attention, awareness, awe, caring, celebration, cherishing, concern, connectedness, curiosity, delight, enjoyment, enthusiasm, interest, intimacy, joy, liking, oneness, peace, regard, respect, responsiveness, sensitivity, surrender, tenderness, thankfulness, warmth, wonder.

BOX 1.2 ACTIVITY

Think about times when you have experienced some of Andrew's heartwarm-ings as shown above. Take a piece of paper and on one side write: *times I have experienced connectedness*. Take your time with this and call to mind your memories of feeling connected to someone or something. Feel free to relive special moments that you think about, recall where you were and what was happening. You will find it a positive and heart-warming experience, just think-ing about it.

Next, pick one of the words and go and experience it now. For example, you could choose *thankfulness*. Go and find something or someone you are thank-ful for: examples could be your legs, your grocery delivery person, your friends, your comfortable bed. Take a minute or two to have the experience of thankfulness.

When you have taken a few minutes to complete the activity in Box 1.2, you will see that it is completely within your power to do so. The more you practise experiencing connection or thankfulness or any of the other aspects of loving in Andrew's list, the more you will see that you do not have to wait for some-thing or someone rare and incredibly special to come along to practise an aspect of loving. Although very special things can happen, it will drastically reduce your opportunities for loving if you are waiting for that, and this is not good, because being loving makes *you* feel good! Andrew's *heartwarmings* show us that we all have love within us and can become experts at loving. It is rewarding and you can develop it like any other skill.

In midwifery care, we can practise and develop these different aspects of loving in many different ways. Part II of this book explores different ways of giving loving midwifery care, for example, using touch, actions and words.

Love as a value in healthcare

In his 1984 exploration of the theology of professional care, Campbell points out a fundamental paradox that health and social care professionals are paid to love. The language used in the book feels slightly outdated in the twenty-first century, but he courageously addresses the complexity of the relation-ship between self-interest (receiving a salary, career progression) and altruism. He argued that if love could be understood in its entirety, with all its respon-sibilities and consequences, then professionals who provide consistent care can be seen as *moderators of love*. Campbell went on to outline some of the ways that this love can be demonstrated by healthcare professionals.

These include recognising each individual person and their worth, as well as noticing the injustices they see in their work and drawing these to the attention of those in power. He also encouraged caregivers to remain aware of their values while navigating the complexities inherent in professional care settings (Campbell, 1984).

Values are beliefs that motivate people's actions, and they also serve as a guide for human behaviour. We are familiar with the values that are considered appropriate for healthcare, such as respect and compassion. But what about love? Of all the healthcare professions, it is perhaps nursing that has the most to teach us about love as a value. Several nursing theorists and scholars have emphasised the importance of love and common humanity as a core value in nursing practice, including Patricia Benner (2010), Kristen Swanson (Duprey, 2022) and one of the most important nursing theorists: Jean Watson. Watson's theory of caring in nursing (Watson, 1979, 1985, 1996, 2004) emphasises the importance of human connection, empathy and compassion in the nurse–patient relationship. Her theory has been widely used in nurse education to teach students about the importance of humanistic care and the *therapeutic use of self* in nursing practice. She views love as a transformative force that promotes healing, facilitates growth and enhances wellbeing for both patients and nurses. Watson sees love in nursing as a deep connection and concern for the patient. This love is expressed through understanding, compassion and providing holistic care.

While there is evidence that nursing, as a profession, accepts love as a value and that many nurses do accept that their work is underpinned by love (Goldin, 2019), until now there has been limited evidence of this in midwifery. Yet surely love can be a value to underpin midwifery work. Many would say that it already is but that it is just not acknowledged.

Love is a driving force for compassion and authentic caring relationships and can enhance the quality of care provided by midwives. Using love as a value compels us to act with integrity, respecting both the uniqueness of each person and the interconnectedness of all people. Moreover, it can have a positive impact on the midwives themselves. However, it is not without its challenges, for example, when loving values conflict with institutional policies or societal expectations.

Conclusions

This chapter has explored love from many different perspectives – from the historical and religious background; its relationship with compassion, connection and spirituality; and from a philosophical stance. The physiological and evolutionary aspects of this profound human experience were explored as was its link to attachment. After looking at love through a psychological lens, the concept of love as something we *do* was considered and finally set in the context of a value or guide to practise in healthcare, including midwifery. Love is clearly important to reproduction and survival and yet it is so much more. It has been argued that the love between baby and mother (or other primary caregiver) is the blueprint for all other forms of love. Although many different types of love have been described, it has been suggested that one thing that all types of love have in common is that it enables someone to see another's value or special worth. Surely this is an ideal basis for humanised, individualised midwifery care.

Love manifests as both a verb (a choice, a driving action) and a deeply held value that guides decision-making and relationships. But while it has been examined through various lenses, above all, love is deeply personal. This chapter has presented a brief tour of some of the different ways that we might analyse love and some of the ways in which it relates to childbirth, midwives and midwifery. However ultimately, it is personal experience which makes love real. Therefore, it is now time to consider what it means for each and every one of us in relation to our lives and our work in maternity care.

References

Andrews, F. (2010). *The Art and Practice of loving: Living a Heartfelt Yes*. (25th Anniversary ed.). Magic. http://www.heartfeltyes.com/read/

Asadollah, F., Nikfarid, L., Sabery, M., Varzeshnejad, M., & Hashemi, F. (2023). The Impact of Loving-Kindness Meditation on Compassion Fatigue of Nurses Working in the Neonatal Intensive Care Unit: A Randomized Clinical Trial Study. *Holistic Nursing Practice*, *37*(4), 215–222. https://doi.org/10.1097/HNP.0000000000000590

Aydin Kartal, Y., Kaya, L., Yazici, S., Engin, B., & Karakus, R. (2022). Effects of Skin-to-Skin Contact on Afterpain and Postpartum Hemorrhage: A Randomized Controlled Trial. *Nursing & health sciences*, *24*(2), 479–486. https://doi.org/10.1111/nhs.12945

Benner, P. (2010, November 12). *What are your core values that keep you going? What is your true north?* [Video]. IHI Open School. https://www.youtube.com/watch?v=J7_Hgn3DFTQ

Bin Mohammed, G. (2019). *Love and the Holy Qur'an*, (8th ed.). The Islamic Texts Society.

Bowlby, J. (1997). *Attachment and Loss*. (Volume 1: attachment). Pimlico.

Brown, B. (2021). *Atlas of the Heart. Mapping Meaningful Connection and the Language of Human Experience*. Vermilion.

Buckley, S. J. (2015). Executive Summary of Hormonal Physiology of Childbearing: Evidence and Implications for Women, Babies, and Maternity Care. *The Journal of perinatal education*, *24*(3), 145–153. https://doi.org/10.1891/1058-1243.24.3.145

Burunat, E. (2016). Love Is not an Emotion. *Psychology*, *7*(14), 1883. https://doi.org/10.4236/psych.2016.714173

Buss, D. (2018). The Evolution of Love in Humans. in: R.J. Sternberg & K. Sternberg (Eds.), *The New Psychology of Love* (4th ed., pp. 42–63). Cambridge University Press.

Byrom, S., Ménage, D., & Patterson, J. (in print). Compassion as a Cure - Humanising Midwifery Work. In E. Newnham, L. McKellar, Mayra, K., & Kuipers, K. (Eds.), *Humanising Birth - Solutions for the Global Maternity Crisis*. Springer Nature.

Campbell, A. (1984). *Moderated Love: A Theology of Professional Care*. SPCK.

Chen, H., Liu, C., Cao, X., Hong, B., Huang, D. H., Liu, C. Y., & Chiou, W. K. (2021). Effects of Loving-Kindness Meditation on Doctors' Mindfulness, Empathy, and Communication Skills. *International Journal of Environmental Research and Public Health*, *18*(8), 4033. https://doi.org/10.3390/ijerph18084033

De Dreu, C. K. W. (2016). Oxytocin Conditions Human Group Psychology. In E. Harmon-Jones & M. Inzlicht (Eds.), *Social Neuroscience: Biological Approaches to Social Psychology* (pp. 143–163). Routledge/Taylor & Francis Group. https://doi.org/10.4324/9781315628714-8

Duprey, K. (2022, November 14). *Kirsten Swanson's Theory of Caring Presentation* [Video]. PechaKucha. https://www.pechakucha.com/presentations/kristins-presentation-892

Fromm, E. (1956). *The Art of Loving*. Harper & Row.

Gilbert, P. (2017). Compassion: Definitions and Controversies. In P. Gilbert (Ed.), *Compassion: Concepts, Research and Applications* (pp. 3–15). Routledge.

Goldin, M. (2019). Nursing as Love: A Hermeneutical Phenomenological Study of Creative Thought Within Nursing. *International Journal for Human Caring*, *23*(4), 312–319. https://doi.org/10.20467/1091-5710.23.4.312

Greenstock, K. (2023). *Flourish; A Practical and Emotional Guidebook to Thriving in Midwifery*. Pinter and Martin Ltd..

Hatfield, E. (1989). Passionate and Compassionate Love. In R. J. Stenberg, & M. L. Barnes (Eds.), *The Psychology of Love* (pp. 191–217). Yale University Press.

Helm, B. (2021). Love. In E.N. Zalta (Ed.), *The Stanford Encyclopedia of Philosophy* (Fall ed.). https://plato.stanford.edu/archives/fall2021/entries/love

hooks, b. (2001). *All About Love: New Visions*. Harper Collins.

Karimi, F. Z., Heidarian Miri, H., Salehian, M., Khadivzadeh, T., & Bakhshi, M. (2019). The Effect of Mother-Infant Skin to Skin Contact after Birth on Third Stage of Labor: A Systematic Review and Meta-Analysis. *Iranian journal of public health*, *48*(4), 612–620. https://www.ncbi.nlm.nih.gov/pmc/articles/PMC6500522/#:~:text=Conclusion%3A,of%20third%20stage%20of%20labor

King, M. L. (1963). *I Have a Dream. Full Speech*. [Video]. YouTube. https://www.youtube.com/watch?v=bNBGvaSHWbY

Lephard, E. (2024). No More 'Us' and 'Them'. *The Practising Midwife*, *27*(5), 29–31. https://doi.org/10.55975/CZMU3005

Longrich, N. R. (2020). *The Origin and Evolution of Love. The Conversation*. https://theconversation.com/the-origin-and-evolution-of-love-131109#:~:text=But%20we're%20hard%2Dwired,the%20time%20of%20the%20dinosaurs

Marazziti, D., Palermo, S., & Mucci, F. (2021). The Science of Love: State of the Art. *Advances in Experimental Medicine and Biology*, *1331*, 249–254. https://doi.org/10.1007/978-3-030-74046-7_16

May, V. (2011). Self, Belonging and Social Change. *Sociology*, *45*(3), 363–378. https://doi.org/10.1177/0038038511399624

Medaris, A. J. (2018). *The State of Falling in Love*. [Doctoral Thesis]. William James College. Proquest. https://www.proquest.com/docview/2076440064

Menage, D., Bailey, E., Lees, S., & Coad, J. (2020). Women's Lived Experience of Compassionate Midwifery: Human and Professional. *Midwifery*, *85*, 102662. https://doi.org/10.1016/j.midw.2020.102662

Mercado, F. (2023). Bridging Divides: Understanding and Overcoming "Othering" Unraveling the Fabric of Othering for an Inclusive and Empathetic World. *Psychology Today*. https://www.psychologytoday.com/intl/blog/the-authentic-self/202312/bridging-divides-understanding-and-overcoming-othering

Mercer, L., Cookson, A., Simpson-Adkins, G., & van Vuuren, J. (2023). Prevalence of Adverse Childhood Experiences and Associations With Personal and Professional Factors in Health and Social Care Workers: A Systematic Review. *Psychological Trauma: Theory, Research, Practice and Policy, 15*(Suppl 2), S231–S245. https://doi.org/10.1037/tra0001506

Moseley, A. (2023). *The Philosophy of Love Part 2* [Video]. YouTube. https://www.youtube.com/watch?v=Kv2dAEgHtLQ

Neff, K. (2011). *Self-Compassion: The Proven Power of Being Kind to Yourself.* William Morrow.

Plummer, J. (2023, June 21). *The Transformational Power of Love in Hinduism: Uma Viswanathan's Perspective on Love in Hinduism.* https://www.templeton.org/news/the-transformational-power-of-love-in-hinduism

Rakhshani, Z. (2017). The Golden Rule and its Consequences: A Practical and Effective Solution for World Peace. *Journal of History Culture and Art Research, 6*(1), 465–473. https://api.semanticscholar.org/CorpusID:151321043

Salzberg, S. (2011). Mindfulness and Loving-Kindness. *Contemporary Buddhism, 12*(1), 177–182. https://doi.org/10.1080/14639947.2011.564837

Saxton, A., Fahy, K., Rolfe, M., Skinner, V., & Hastie, C. (2015). Does Skin-to-Skin Contact and Breast Feeding at Birth Affect the Rate of Primary Postpartum Haemorrhage: Results of a Cohort Study. *Midwifery, 31*(11), 1110–1117. https://doi.org/10.1016/j.midw.2015.07.008

Schwartz, R. & Olds, J. (2015). *Love and the Brain.* Harvard Medical School.

Scott Peck, M. (2002). *The Road Less Travelled* (25th Anniversary ed.). Simon and Shuster.

Seidman, J. (2009). Valuing and Caring. *Theoria, 75*(4), 272–303. https://www.researchgate.net/publication/227843360_Valuing_and_Caring#fullTextFileContent

Sheth, N. (2006). Christian and Buddhist Altruistic Love. *Gregorianum, 87*(4), 810–826. http://www.jstor.org/stable/23581627

The New Revised Standard Version Bible. (1995). Oxford University Press.

The Orthodox Jewish Bible. (2011). Artists for Israel International. https://www.afii.org/OJB.pdf

Walter, M. H., Abele, H., & Plappert, C. F. (2021). The Role of Oxytocin and the Effect of Stress During Childbirth: Neurobiological Basics and Implications for Mother and Child. *Frontiers in Endocrinology, 12*, 742236. https://doi.org/10.3389/fendo.2021.742236

Watson, J. (1979). *Nursing. The Philosophy and Science of Caring.* Little, Brown and Co. Revised (1985, 1991, 2008) University Press of Colorado.

Watson, J. (1985). *Nursing: Human Science and Human Care. A Theory of Nursing.* Appleton and Lange. Reprinted (1988) National League for Nursing Press, (1999, 2007). Jones and Bartlett.

Watson, J. (1996). Watson's Theory of Transpersonal Caring. In: P. H. Walker & B. Newman (Eds.), *Blueprint for Use of Nursing Models: Education, Research, Practice and Administration* (pp. 141–153). National League for Nursing.

Watson, J. (2004). *Caring Science as Sacred Science.* F. A. Davis Company.

Watson, T., Watts, L., Waters, R., & Hodgson, D. (2023). The Benefits of Loving Kindness Meditation for Helping Professionals: A Systematic Review. *Health & Social Care in the Community, 2023*(3),1–14. https://doi.org/10.1155/2023/5579057

Young, E. S., Simpson, J. A., Griskevicius, V., Huelsnitz, C. O., & Fleck, C. (2019). Childhood Attachment and Adult Personality: A Life History Perspective. *Self and Identity, 18*(1), 22–38. https://doi.org/10.1080/15298868.2017.1353540

2

LOVE AND THE HUMANISATION OF CHILDBIRTH

Lesley Page and Clare Wardhaugh

Hello Dear Reader,

We are so happy to have you read our letters about love, midwifery, and humanising childbirth.

These letters form a conversation between Lesley Page, an experienced midwife who has worked to humanise childbirth over many years, and Clare Wardhaugh. Clare, through her work in education, person-centred counselling and embodied spiritual direction, has enabled practitioners to authentically practise personal beliefs in their workplace with integrity, critical thinking, and values of love.

In writing these letters, we are thinking about you. What is your life like? We wonder what you think about the idea that love is the key to humanising childbirth. We wonder what your work is like. Have you had a good day or a bad day at work? Do you work in an organisation? If so, is it one that helps you give of your best, or one that makes it more difficult?

Whatever your circumstances, we hope our exploration from our different perspectives will illuminate the importance of love to our lives, and love in midwifery practice. The start of life, pregnancy, labour, and birth, and the early weeks of life is a critical and sensitive period in which the transcendent growth of love, attachment, and strong family relationships may be supported, or disturbed. Midwifery is vital to ensuring that the growth of love and commitment is supported rather than undermined at the start of life.

We hope that through reading this conversation, midwives and others will be inspired to think about what love means and reflect on the place of love in their lives, their practice, and in the systems and cultures in which they work.

With our warmest regards
Lesley and Clare

DOI: 10.4324/9781032645780-4

Dear Lesley,

I have often pondered on how love manifests itself in life. In my life I must face my own sense of failure and disappointment that I have not lived up to the beliefs and vision I have for my own practice of love.

I say this because when reading about the theory and practice of love, I become both inspired and despondent at the same time, thinking I can never attain such high ideals. However, I must always remember it is progress not perfection that I strive for. The theory of love is our touchstone, something that informs and drives our visions and beliefs, but the reality of practising love is very complex.

To start our letters, I thought it might be helpful to clarify the love of which I speak. Our English language is limited when it comes to love. Love covers many expressions from, "I love chocolate" to "I love my child." However, these require a different depth and intensity of response.

Lesley, I understand concepts in a very visual way, and so, when I think about love, the image that means most to me is that of a diamond. The diamond is a useful image, as a diamond radiates different colours from its many facets. So, although it is one substance, it illuminates many different qualities into the world.

So, with love, we can talk about kindness, compassion, generosity, gentleness, strength, care, empathy, and courage, all being expressed in the world, through the varied facets of that one beautiful concept, love. Love is an intentional relational energy. Love only exists in the world when experienced in a relationship, like that of a mother, child, and midwife. Love is a sensory experience, it cannot exist in the mind only, it must be embodied. Through our senses, we intuit a presence, we feel a touch, we hear a tone of voice, we see a face, all of which feeds into our understanding of whether we are in the presence of love or not. So, what affects our human capacity to love?

We are embodied people. We exist in this world and are connected to the energies that exist in the cosmos. We can see in our embodied self, how the energies that exist within us exist and indeed are mirrored in the cosmos. The universe creates environments that allow life and different potential, to develop and expand. So, with humans, we have the capacity to create environments that allow for growth and life. However, within the cosmos lies the energy of black holes. They have the potential to suck in life, so that eventually the gravitational pull is so great that there is no resisting, and all life is pulled in, stretched, destroyed, and drawn into nothingness.

Love is the difference between a life-giving or life-taking environment. By this I do not mean physical life or death, but emotional, psychological, spiritual, and intellectual life or death.

Pierre Teilhard de Chardin (a Christian theologian of the 20th century) says that

> Human love is the energy that drives whatever we do to keep ourselves and our world growing together in unity and peace...Helping the human family move toward the next step of evolution in love is the most urgent and challenging task of contemporary spirituality.
>
> *(Savary & Berne, 2017, pp. 3,5)*

We can choose to use this love energy in relationships to give life and offer the development of full potential to others and ourselves or, we can choose to offer destruction and nothingness. As individuals and institutions, we can choose to create or destroy, and this can be done consciously or unconsciously. So surely love must be understood as an intentional act of energy that provides the conditions in which we ourselves and others can grow in our humanity towards our life's purpose. Do our actions in the workplace and life relationships create an environment that gives life to people where they can experience safety, kindness, knowledge, goodness, and caring, and where self-worth and self-esteem and occupational and relational skills are developed? Or do we, through our actions, create an environment where we disregard, criticise, judge, and belittle, thus destroying self-worth and self-esteem which detract from confidence in practising occupational skills? Many of us will have worked in *black hole institutions*, where we are stretched beyond recognition and drawn into emptiness and professional destruction by the systems and bureaucracy in place. In most faith traditions, it is considered sacred to follow the drive to resist this destructive energy, in us and institutions, and to work towards the common good for all.

Our capacity to love is affected by our experience of love. We either imitate or rebel against our experience, and at times the imitation is not based on a healthy understanding and practice of love. This in turn affects the people with whom we are in contact, positively or negatively. It is important therefore to have the skills to reflect on how our particular personhood impacts on others and whether that fits with the institution's mission statements. It is important to recognise that we are born with a unique DNA mix; our mix has never existed before in the world and will never exist again. The child born offers a specific and unique gift to creation. Their uniqueness is sacred and unless their giftedness is nurtured, their unique purpose is lost to all humanity forever. I believe it is our responsibility to create an environment where this potential and purpose can be developed.

I will leave it there for now Lesley,

Much love

Clare

Dear Clare,

When I got your letter, I was struck by your image of love as a diamond, with its different facets, sparkling in different colours. Midwives are surrounded by this life-giving energy, or at least its potential, in all their work. The time around birth is a critical start to our capacity to love, and for each baby being born, and their parents, to offer their own specific and unique gift to creation and fulfil their unique purpose.

You talk about our responsibility to create an environment where the purpose and potential of each child can be developed. The time around birth is critical to a life in which the child being born, and the mother, father, or other parent may each reach their potential. To know about the love we talk about.

For many years, I have worked with Soo Downe, Jane Sandall, and Carmen Power to humanise childbirth. Humanising childbirth is a phrase that is heard frequently. It can mean different things to different people. It is, like your love diamond, multi-dimensional. In our definition, the recognition of the infinite possibilities of the life that lies ahead of the baby being born, and the potential for love and social thriving must be supported. We wrote,

> Childbirth (the period around pregnancy, labour and birth and the early weeks of life) is a time of promise and potential. It is a time of infinite possibilities, with the potential for love and social thriving, as well as for optimal health and wellbeing. The consequences can resonate beyond the short term, over a lifetime, and into the next generation. There is hope for a better chance in life. Humanising childbirth helps keep the promise and fulfil the potential of the mother and child. If childbirth is humanised, it can stimulate positive transformative neurohormonal, physical and psychosocial effects of pregnancy, labour, birth, and early life for individuals, the family, community, and wider society.

It is strange that in a world where we talk about love so often, and that in midwifery where we see love manifest in behaviour and feelings every day, love is rarely discussed explicitly. While much of my writing has been implicitly about love around childbirth and in midwifery, I am now surprised how little I used the word.

Yet love is vital to the future of our world and society, and the human race – love of others, by others, love of our mother earth, and her resources. As you quote, Teilhard de Chardin says our most urgent and challenging life's purpose is to transform the world through helping the human family grow in love.

Clare, my mind is racing as I read your letter, moving from the embodiment and manifestation of love. How do we move from the high principles described by Teilhard de Chardin to the down-to-earth, complicated, often messy business of childbirth and those exhausting weeks of early life. How does love grow as life is turned upside down when this new precious life enters the world, and the parents, especially the mother, experience a profound metamorphosis with physical and emotional change? How are the woman becoming mother, the other parent, the new family, supported to transcend these challenges, so that through love for their baby, they experience joy and delight, even in the exhaustion and confusion?

We are talking with midwives, and others responsible for providing the best care around childbirth. How do they recognise and support this journey that enhances and magnifies the positive energy of love in all its manifestations?

Childbirth is a critical and sensitive period where love can be supported, so the newborn is cherished, and the baby, mother, and family may be helped to thrive, rather than just survive. Optimal physical and mental health, alongside prevention of harm, of the baby, mother, and family, are critical to sensitive, responsive, competent, and confident parenting.

Perhaps first we need an awareness of the importance of a secure attachment between the baby and the primary caregiver (usually the mother), and the family, to short- and long-term health, happiness, and future relationships. In this first love relationship of life, the baby, held by the mother or parent, may experience being held in love for the first time. We need to recognise that this love or attachment may be supported or blocked and disturbed, by individuals and institutions, by circumstances. How may midwives, other professionals, birth workers, and institutions strengthen this attachment? A concern to strengthen this attachment enhances and does not limit healthcare. The greatest challenge may be how we provide for these unique people, the baby being born and the parents, either in industrial healthcare systems designed for the greatest throughput of people at the lowest cost or private services designed to make a profit. I would love to know what you think about this, the nature of care around childbirth strengthening rather than weakening the bonds of love, the commitment that comes from the attachment.

You rightly ask if I think birth is sacred, and you talk about the unique human being coming into existence. Of course, but when I think of something sacred it seems a bit other worldly. What I know is that this human being will never be born again. This human being is on the threshold of life, a world of potential. There is the chance to create environments that allow for growth and life.

As you so eloquently put it, love is manifest in the body, so yes, birth is both sacred and earthly.

This is probably enough for today, except to say I think many of those reading this will feel there are no true choices for us to create spaces of positive energy and avoid the black holes. Life circumstances, the nature of our institutions and governments, may enhance or limit our choices, our human potential. The world around us now grappling with enormous jumps in technical ability without the wisdom to manage it, the terrible wars that continue, the dystopian politics, all limit potential.

Yet still I believe that if we get birth right, we will contribute enormously to a better world. This is the basis of humanising childbirth.

Perhaps hope is an essential element of love? What do you think?

Love

Lesley

Dear Lesley,

Thank you so much for your wonderful letter.

Midwifery, where love is first experienced and yes, hope ignited. This made me consider how important it is to make that first contact positive so as to nurture the holistic development of mother, child, and parent.

In that first experience of love, I can intuit the holistic vulnerability of the moment, where that positive contact can be embraced or lost. Vulnerability is surely one of the gateway emotions which can lead to love. Vulnerability, such a fragile part of our humanity, can be received with care, attention, professional knowledge, dignity, and respect, which leads to the growth of self-esteem and self-worth, *or* it cannot. Vulnerability makes us feel powerless. In our powerlessness, we need someone to meet the need of our impotence. Love is that power. Love is manifest in the world through people. So, the *other* we need in our vulnerability can be a midwife who is a conduit for that loving relational power to flow through them to the other, allowing the vulnerability to be met with graciousness, promoting dignity and understanding which are important ingredients for the growth of love.

Lesley, you wrote about how we shy away from the word love, in so many professions, but particularly in midwifery. Perhaps we are afraid of this word. Fear because it can be an energy that exposes our own lack of understanding or experience and can lead to a feeling of vulnerability, which is both threatening and uncomfortable for professionals to feel. Perhaps this could be addressed in midwifery training or continuous professional development (CPD) so that comfort can be encouraged, and fear dispelled. Love can be difficult to talk about and that may be because we live in an age where there is an expectation that everything is evidenced and measured.

But why do we want to evidence and measure love? And in the attempt to do this, do we then control and formalise this action, the end result being that a spontaneous and creative energy, which should be freely exercised with competence and responsibility, is suffocated and dampened. When talking of the practice of love in an institution, I think that this point needs to be considered.

In a professional setting, love is often understood as a *soft action*, someone who is meek, mild, and nice. Like the Jesus image that has been promoted historically and which has influenced, in particular, our western mentality and culture, and has also influenced how the progression of our health and educative institutions have evolved. However, if Jesus was meek and mild and nice, why was he eventually publicly executed for political and religious agitation? So, we need to move away from the image of love as a *soft option* and reclaim the concept that love is a strong action which demands discipline and commitment, dedication and intentional action which at times needs courage, but always needs the practice of consistency and reflection.

Carl Rogers (psychologist) developed the qualities which need to exist in professional relationships for a true therapeutic and transformative experience to happen. He speaks of positive regard, empathy, and congruence as being the ingredients that need to be present in the relationship for change and remodelling to develop (Rogers, 1957). How, Lesley, does this apply in midwifery? When you spoke about childbirth as being the time of promise and potential, I saw the difference between my understanding of transformation and transfiguration. That precious childbirth time can be seen as one of transformation, where the child, parents, and midwives change and become something new. Or we can see childbirth as a time where the child, parents, and midwives transfigure to become and grow closer to the people they were born to be, and in this way, fulfilling the potential of which you speak. One speaks of change and the other speaks of fulfilment. Fulfilment, I think, connects more with your idea of promise and potential. If the correct conditions exist, then we can each become *more ourselves as a midwife, more ourselves as a parent* and the child is given the inviting conditions to become their self.

The love attachment is, of course, better experienced as early as possible, but, as we have discussed, it is not always the case for all babies to experience this perfection during childbirth and those exhausting first weeks. It is important though not to lose hope. We must never forget the innate capacity born uniquely in each one of us to develop into who we are meant to be as loving humans, contributing positively with our own unique gifts and talents to the world.

Carl Rogers (1957) speaks about the actualising tendency present in each human. He compares it to potatoes! If a potato is left in a cupboard without the natural conditions present to allow for its healthy growth, the actualising tendency of the potato will still strive to grow towards whatever light there is. It may end up being a misshapen version of its true self but the drive to actualise itself and its primary purpose will not be subdued. This is true of humans' actualising tendencies. Most will find our way towards our true self. If the loving conditions are not present from our primary caregivers, we may end up distorted in our growth. However, this actualising tendency is so strong in us that it will always look for the light of love to grow towards. This may be met in nursery, school, relationships, professions, and healing professions, anywhere.

So, as you said, humanising midwifery through love is about care. However, what values and energies drive and sustain midwives to consistently offer this loving care? What should exist to overcome the despondency, fatigue, disillusionment, and fear so that positive loving and hopeful environments can be offered? How can the institutions ensure that this type of environment exists to nurture midwives?

I will leave it there for now Lesley, wishing you much love,

Clare

Dear Clare,

I have been rereading your early letters and thinking about our conversations. I was pulled back to the work of Michel Odent, a French obstetrician and childbirth specialist. I have known and talked with Michel over many years particularly about his primal health research. Much of what you say chimes with his work, especially his book: *The Scientification of Love* (Odent, 1999). Michel underlines the utmost importance of the development of the capacity to love, love in its broadest sense. The vital lessons of the book are

...that of all the different manifestations of love: maternal, paternal, filial, sexual, romantic, platonic, spiritual, brotherly, not to mention love of country, love of inanimate objects, and compassion and concern for Mother Earth. The prototype of all these ways of loving is maternal love.

(Odent, 1999, p. 2)

This links with what I wrote earlier about childbirth being a short, critical, sensitive period in which this capacity to love in the baby, mother, parent, and family, may be enhanced, or reduced, and the vital role midwives have in this. Michel wrote about how the nature of love and how the capacity to love develops, have become subjects of scientific study, with implications at least as important as those of genetics, electronics, or quantum theory. Michel envisions that when we learn to harness the energies of love, this will be as pivotal as the discovery of fire, although some see this as utopian.

You Clare have provided an essential theology, philosophy, and understanding of love. Love is an intentional act of energy that provides the conditions in which we can all grow in our humanity towards our life's purpose. So, you and Michel both draw on the work of Teilhard de Chardin.

Michel sees human evolution in love as an evolutionary shift. The next step in this shift, I believe, is long overdue. Current sciences indicate that the capacity to love is a prerequisite for long term and global survival, to thrive with emotional and physical wellbeing. A dominant concern to develop a capacity to love, which includes love for our environment and mother earth, may help the survival of humanity and protection of, and equal accessibility to, the earth's resources.

Yet, there remains strong resistance to the need to enhance the capacity of the baby, the woman becoming mother, and the family to love. Why? Michel believes that the extreme specialisation of sciences means that most scientists, including the medical profession, seem unaware of the science around this. Like when a brightly shining mirror is full of cracks making it difficult to see the whole. More than this, the science is not considered mainstream, or politically correct, being largely ignored and denied. The evidence base for the physiology, biological changes, and neurohormonal effect that helps prime the woman for mothering is seen as contentious and is often decried and denigrated.

Again, why? Supporting a firm foundation in a strong bond of love, and secure attachments, will not interfere in the safety of birth. The converse is true. Supporting the complex biological processes of childbirth underlies health, wellbeing, and secure attachments.

When these biological mechanisms are disturbed, we must understand how compensation may be made. Many things disturb these biological mechanisms, such as: pathology (the biological mechanisms not working, no homeostasis) requiring perhaps induction of labour, caesarean section, and epidural; fear or extreme anxiety, or traumatic experience; or perhaps unsympathetic birth workers or disrespectful care.

Resistance to the theories and concepts, the practices that support development of the capacity to love, and of secure attachments, are deeply rooted in culture, embedded routines, and set ways of thinking about childbirth. The energy of this resistance is strong. It seems to me that there is a huge defence mechanism at play, preventing an acceptance of the sciences that are so important to our future. Those who wish to disseminate this science and its implications are often silenced. I see this defence in individuals as well as in organisations, leaders of professions, influencers, and the media. In the United Kingdom, it pervades the culture around childbirth.

Perhaps because, as many of us feel, we regret that we didn't know as much when we raised our children, and that we might have done better. Perhaps because we ourselves did not experience the love, security, and care that we needed. Perhaps we have had extremely traumatic experiences.

How then can midwives, who have a vitally important role, support rather than undermine the conditions in which mothers, and their babies in particular, the other parent, and family, may grow in their capacity to love? How can they set them on a path to lifelong emotional and physical wellbeing? I think, as a profession, we must understand that our care around childbirth, as Michel tells us, has long-term consequences for the development of the capacity to love, which we ignore at our peril.

My friend and colleague Barbara Mills, a child psychotherapist, and I wrote what I believe was the first midwifery book chapter to have the word love in its title: *The Growth of Human Love and Commitment* (Mills & Page, 2000). We wrote, "The human infant's attachment to the mother (or other primary caregiver) is a prerequisite for survival and a test bed for all other attachments that he or she will have in the future" (p. 223). Also, that importantly, the midwife "is a facilitator not only of the physical birth, but also of the birth of the self, the family and the potential for human love" (p. 223).

This birth of the self is profound. You wrote earlier about transfiguration and may, I think, have something more to say about this. A person's own experience of being parented is a key influence on their future parenting style and behaviour. Also, the period around childbirth is vitally important where positive parenting can be established, and cycles of negative parenting, abuse and neglect can be broken. This is a time of extreme neuroplasticity in the brain of the baby, and intense openness particularly in the woman becoming mother, but in the partner and family too.

The midwife is well placed to support parents in developing positive parenting. This is especially valuable when the ability to parent positively is at risk through life history or other factors. The woman who is traumatised, ill, or suffering mental health problems will find it difficult to practise love, to provide the sensitive responses that her baby needs. To enable midwives in this support, systems of care must promote optimal health, wellbeing, and happiness in the long and short term.

This is more possible when midwives can build relationships of trust with women, particularly if this starts early in pregnancy and, through continuity, is built over time. Then the midwife may, through her sensitive responses to the woman's needs, provide an experience that the mother may in turn, provide for her baby. Through such trust, the midwife may encourage the parents to reflect on their experience of being parented, what they value, and what they would change. The midwife can also ensure that mother and baby are not separated unnecessarily, that skin to skin care is offered and supported, and that breast feeding is supported. Midwives can help women understand the implications of disturbing complex biological changes, and so enable their decision making. This will need not only *loving practice* by midwives and others, but also, effective care, i.e. care that works. Effective care exists through alternative pathways that allow individual care for women, their babies and families. Such *loving practice* and effective care offer a strong foundation for secure loving relationships, health, and wellbeing in both the short and long term, as well as the potential to thrive, not just survive.

Stoodley and Power (in print) explore, through a comprehensive review of current evidence, the importance of the individual experience of transition to parenthood, support for bonding, and a secure attachment, for a humanised society. The aim is that a newborn infant can hope not just to survive, but crucially to thrive and flourish. It will provide a critical resource to midwives and others.

Clare, I would love to know your responses to this very particular discussion about love, and its central importance to midwives. We need, I think, a different way of thinking about, talking about love. It has been so good to talk with you about love in our letters, and to see it through your eyes.

With love for now

Lesley

Dear Lesley,

I am so sad that this will be my last letter to you. You speak so powerfully about love in practice and the need for alternative pathways, effective systems of care, etc., to be found in midwifery.

The history of humankind has long been involved in the quest to find out how to love fruitfully, creating loving communities where we can evolve as individuals and societies. Over many centuries, this spiritual seeking, by all religions, has left us with a wealth of knowledge and disciplines, which, if practised, can help us to live healthy lives of love.

One of the main focuses that most religions and spiritual ways accept is to acknowledge an individual's responsibility to contribute to the wellbeing of society, so that both individuals and societies can grow and evolve in knowledge, empathy, and critical consciousness – a place where the intellectual, the emotional, the spiritual, and the physical aspects of our humanity will be cared for as a whole. I see the individual midwife holding the responsibility for this care at the crucial time of birth. Like a stone dropped in a still lake, the ripple effects from that one action of the midwife will expand, touching so many others for good or ill. However, the institution is also responsible to the midwife to ensure that they are being offered, in justice, the opportunity for their own holistic health, growth, and safety.

Just as Carl Rogers offers the core conditions as a way for a therapeutic relationship to evolve, so an institution needs to understand how to create an environment where the conditions for a holistic care of the practitioners and patients is offered. To be an individual or institution where:

> Love is always patient and kind, love is never jealous, love is not boastful or conceited, it is never rude and never seeks its own advantage, it does not take offence or store up grievances. Love does not rejoice at wrongdoing but finds its joy in the truth. It is always ready to make allowances, to trust, to hope and to endure whatever comes. Love never comes to an end.
>
> *(King James Bible, 1769/2019, 1 Corinthians 13:4–8)*

To progress to this, it would be necessary to consider our own, or our institution's, egos, so that they do not negatively affect this environment, and so that this pure strong love can flow freely through us and our institutions to others. This may be a utopian dream, but one which, we as individuals and institutions, could aspire to in the knowledge that it is progress not perfection that we desire. This is the strong love that I spoke of earlier and to honestly live these qualities, awareness needs to be given to where our ego interferes with these qualities of love evolving.

Most religions, disciplines, and philosophies would conclude that awareness is the starting point of how to live loving action. In Buddhism, we would have the practice of mindfulness, where awareness of how we act is observed, where we notice our intentions, and how we manifest all of this is brought to awareness through meditation and mindful actions. In Christianity, there would be the practice of the Sacrament of the present moment, where we are called to be aware of God in that moment and where our actions, thoughts, and intentions are to be in keeping with the values of Christ. In Buddhism, Christianity, and the other major religions, the aim is to act with holistic integrity, so that there is no dissonance between what we believe, what we intend, and how we act. This, of course, takes lifelong learning and demands fearless honesty and a willingness to change. One of the most dynamic contributions to spiritual living in the last and this century is the practical Alcoholics Anonymous (AA) 12 step programme (AA, 2024). Richard Rohr (a Christian theologian) notes, "We are all addicts" (Rohr, 2011, p. xxii). Human beings are addictive by nature. Addiction is a modern name and honest description for what the biblical tradition called *sin* and mediaeval Christians called *passions* or *attachments*. Both AA and Rohr recognised that serious measures or practices were needed to break us out of these illusions and entrapments. The AA programme offers a step-by-step guide as to how to live a life of integrity and authenticity without the need to act out of our addictions, whatever they are, and it provides a community to support the lifelong growth of each individual and their sense of awareness. This fearless honesty, awareness, and willingness to change is an invitation to both the individual and the institution to create a learning environment. One that is committed to real change that is brave enough to look at itself and say, this is not working, forgive us, and then create what will work, as evidenced by practitioners.

Learning communities need reflective practice to provide a place of safety where mistakes, misgivings, disillusionment, bullying, and uncertainty can be discussed and the effects of these experiences on practitioners are also considered. In this way, professional competency is addressed as is the toll on our humanity, for it is the toll that the negative experiences can take on us that affect how we act with others. So, to choose not to recognise this aspect of humanising practice through love is to miss out on the most important instrument of all professional practices, which is the human being practising them. Just as the beautiful Stradivarius violin, playing music with harmony and resonance has to be cared for and cherished, so surely does the individual midwife. The midwife is the Stradivarius, playing, with growing expertise, the symphony of birth, and they have to be given the opportunity to be cared for so that they can lovingly care for the people who are given into their care.

Love is the vital ingredient of that care.

Love has to cascade through the institutions through its values, practised for both practitioners and patients alike. There have to be systems of reflection, and compassionate accountability; there has to be a willingness to accept failure, to learn, and to change. Real change (not one on paper only), involving a change of heart, mind, and action is the invitation of desiring a loving practice.

As Pierre Theilhard de Chardin wrote in 1934:

Someday, after mastering the winds, the waves, the tides, and gravity, we shall harness for God the energies of love, and then, for a second time in the history of the world, man will have discovered fire.

(Teilhard de Chardin, 1974, pp. 86–87)

I shall leave it there dear Lesley.

My heart and love are with you in your life's journey.

Love

Clare

Dear Reader,

We have come to the end of our correspondence for now. It is our hope that these letters have allowed you to explore the different perspectives of love and that they illuminate the importance of love in the practice of midwifery. Perhaps they have affirmed knowledge or intuitions which you already have, or perhaps they have challenged you to have a new perspective or understanding.

We hope that these letters will provide a springboard for further conversations, to consider what love is in the practice of midwifery and what to do to make it intentionally manifest. We also hope that we have considered some practical ways to nurture love in the midwife, so that the fullness of their experience can flow strongly to the other, nurturing mother, child, and parent, to the fullness of their lives.

Our last hope is that through the inspiration of this book, you will know the length, breadth, height, and depth of love and will be both drawn to and sustained in the practice of love in midwifery; this beautiful and precious moment of life. Truth can be seen in loving action, and when it is seen and felt, it has an irresistible pull towards its goodness.

May your precious self be allowed to organically grow in that love, so that it becomes irresistible to pass it on in its true form as the diamond of love.

We wish you much love in your life,

Lesley and Clare

References

AA. (2024). *The 12 steps programme*. https://www.alcoholics-anonymous.org.uk/about-aa/what-is-aa/12-steps/

King James Bible. (2019). Christian Art Publishers. (Original work published 1769).

Mills, B. C. & Page, L.A. (2000). The growth of human love and commitment. In L.A. Page (Ed.), *New midwifery: Science and sensitivity in practice* (pp. 223–244). Elsevier Health Sciences.

Odent, M. (1999). *The scientification of love*. Free Association Books.

Rogers, C. R. (1957). The necessary and sufficient conditions of therapeutic personality change. *Journal of Consulting Psychology*, *21*(2), 95–103. https://doi.org/10.1037/h0045357

Rohr, R. (2011). *Breathing under water*. Franciscan Media.

Savary, L.M. & Berne, P.H. (2017). *Teilhard de Chardin on Love: Evolving human relationships*. Paulist press.

Stoodley, C. & Power, C. (in print) Transition to Parenthood, Bonding and Attachment. The keys to humanised society. In E. Newnham, L. McKellar, Mayra, K., & Kuipers, K. (Eds.). *Humanising birth - Solutions for the global maternity crisis*. Springer Nature.

Theilhard de Chardin, P. (1974). The evolution of chastity. In *Toward the future*. Harper Collins. Glasgow. (1936). Online reference: "The Evolution of Chastity". In *Toward the Future*, XI, 86–87. https://teilharddechardin.org/teilhard-de-chardin/teilhards-quotes/

3

WHY WE NEED TO TALK ABOUT LOVE IN MIDWIFERY

Elizabeth Newnham

Introduction

Why is it necessary to be talking about love in midwifery? The most striking thing about maternity care systems, when looking at research and reports of these systems worldwide, is the distinct lack of *care*, and featuring instead obstetric violence and racism, birth trauma, increased mortality for marginalised populations, dysfunctional institutions, and disenfranchised midwives (Davis, 2019; Fleszar et al., 2023; Foster et al., 2024; Newnham et al., 2018; Sadler et al., 2016; Thomas, 2024; Watson et al., 2021; World Health Organization, 2014), and a system of care that does not live up to its name, or its purpose.

How then, do we start to address this situation that appears beyond fixing, that is, the dire absence of care in a system supposedly designed to provide care during a critical, vulnerable, meaningful yet extremely common event in the lives of women, birthing people, their babies, and families?

With this book, bringing love into the equation provides a way to start addressing some of these issues. A deeply human experience, love has tended perhaps to be explored more in poetry and music than in professional discourse. Love has also been left by the wayside in the wake of more prominent tread patterns in our human history, those of violence, war, colonisation, oppression, domination, and control. Love may have also disappeared from view during medicalisation, with the separation of body and mind, of sex and birth, of professional and personal, of clinical and experiential. In this chapter, I first outline the concept of love, then position it as central to relational midwifery care, and to what colleagues and I have recently termed *relational midwifery thinking*, through the practice of attention. I then outline the role of love

DOI: 10.4324/9781032645780-5

and care in political action to argue that love is not only an essential element of quality maternity care, but necessary for reproductive justice.

Theoretical considerations

To support the arguments below, I am drawing on feminist philosopher Sara Ruddick's (1990) thesis on maternal thinking with a focus on her ideas about attentiveness, through a lens of care ethics, for which attention is also central.

Sara Ruddick's work on *maternal thinking* identified the embodied practice of mothering as encouraging a *thinking in practice* that is inherently relational and contextual and identifying the aims of maternal thinking as being preservative love, nurturance, and training for social acceptability. Ruddick then developed maternal thinking as a way to conceptualise a politics and practice of peace, as well as to challenge the Western philosophical construct of *reason*; asking "was it possible to reconceive a reason that strengthened passion rather than opposing it, that refused to separate love from knowledge?" (Ruddick, 1990, p.9). Ruddick sees mothering as a practice rather than a role, so, she argues, the work of *mothering*, although disproportionately gendered, is not inherently biological. Ruddick's ideas about maternal thinking, particularly the focus on relationality and attention, will be drawn on in this chapter in relation to the importance of developing the idea of love in midwifery.

The other theoretical concept I will draw on in this chapter is that of care ethics. Care ethics has grown out of feminist critique of moral and ethical reasoning, and centres care as a praxis (practice and theory) that is grounded in relationality (Newnham & Kirkham, 2019; Tronto, 2020). Care ethics positions *care* as central to human life that "includes everything we do to maintain, contain, and repair our 'world' so that we can live in it as well as possible" (Tronto, 2020, p.103). It is acknowledged that everyone needs care. Tronto's care ethics contains four elements: attentiveness, responsibility, competence, and responsiveness (for more on this, see Newnham & Kirkham, 2019).

While we may think of care as relating only to moments of *caring for*, such as infants, the ill, or the elderly, the positioning of care as central to all life emphasises human interdependency between each other and our environment. Even those who do not appear to need care, still receive it. However, in the late capitalist economy, the exchange of money for *care* conceals this fact. Think of the activities of growing and cooking food. If we are busy, and have enough money, we outsource these activities (e.g., by shopping in the supermarket, going to a restaurant). In this instance, we are receiving care, because someone else is growing or cooking our food. This elemental human need for care opposes the construct of the *individual*, central to the philosophies of late capitalism and neoliberalism, epitomised by privatisation and dismantling of social welfare policies. The perpetuation of the myth that all people are ruggedly self-reliant, and able to achieve all things if they just work hard enough, is central to the overlapping ideologies of capitalism, patriarchy, and colonialism.

What is love?

I will begin with a definition, because in order to talk about a thing, one first needs to know what it is. In bell hook's *All about Love*, she acknowledges how little has been written about love in any serious sense, and uses a definition from M. Scott Peck that love is: "the will to extend oneself for the purpose of nurturing one's own or another's spiritual growth" (hooks, 2017, p. 4). The idea of spiritual growth can be substituted for self-actualisation or human flourishing. Importantly, hooks argues that love is not simply a feeling, an emotion over which we have little or no control (as the poetry and songs may tell us); love is an action, a practice, a choice.

With this meaning understood, there can be clarification of some of the more muddying aspects of love in the context of human relationships, which are complex, and subject to dysfunction. This dysfunction is perhaps unsurprising given that in many parts of the world, people have been trying to thrive within societies that, in the aftereffects of capitalism, patriarchy, and colonialism, prioritise the individual over community, profit over equity, and resources over the environment. Societies underpinned by these values can only exist through exploitation, and the social institutions within them have become increasingly dehumanising. Love – the stretching of oneself to enable another's growth – according to hooks, cannot coexist with abuse. Any relationships that have within them abusive or disrespectful behaviours and that do not consider foremost the flourishing of the other are not loving relationships. Other behaviours may be confused with love, such as caretaking, affection, or interest; however, if these also include abuse of any kind, they cannot, by definition, be loving. Genuine love, according to hooks (2017), is a "combination of care, commitment, trust, knowledge, responsibility, and respect" (pp. 7-8). If one of these six elements is missing, then the presence of love must be questioned.

These six elements are relevant to maternity care providers with respect to relationships of care. The care element is self-explanatory. Commitment and responsibility can be related to a dedication to the profession, to upholding professional standards such as confidentiality and lifelong learning. Responsibility is also one of the key elements of care ethics and relates to being accountable for one's own capacity and capability to undertake caring activities. Knowledge can refer to the professional knowledge base, of basing practice on evidence, as well as self-knowledge (one's own biases and assumptions) and knowledge of the person for whom you are caring. Indeed, we could link this *knowledge* element of love to evidence informed healthcare, the principles of which are to incorporate current evidence, clinical expertise, and experience, and most importantly, the wishes and context of the person making the decision (Sackett et al., 1996).

And finally, the last two elements of love, respect, and trust, are vital in maternity care, and we usually talk about these in terms of developing rapport and building relationships. However, perhaps less examined is the reason why this is so important, not only because of the significance of the pregnancy and birth event, or because respect and trust should be expected in most healthcare provider relationships, but also due to its intimacy as a sexual and reproductive act. Care for the maternal body also involves seeing and touching parts that are usually perceived as private, so not only is the perinatal period emotionally intimate, it is also physically intimate. Given this intimacy, it is perhaps more vital in maternity settings that women are able to trust their care providers, and that care providers understand the magnitude of their responsibility in holding this trust. Not to do so leads to experiences of bodily violation, commonly reported in the literature (see, e.g., Keedle et al., 2024; Mayra et al., 2022). To address this, midwives (and other maternity care providers) need to be absolutely clear on what consent and bodily self-determination actually mean. This is not currently occurring for several reasons, partly because current bioethical frameworks are not sufficient (Newnham & Kirkham, 2019), and partly because systems of care are set up to serve their own ends, rather than actually provide individualised, humanised care (Feeley, 2023; Newnham et al., 2018; Niles et al., 2021; van der Waal et al., 2021).

Trust is also eroded through coercion or the giving of skewed or misinformation (Buchanan et al., 2023). hooks (2017) notes that any form of lying (including withholding information) impinges on love, while recognising that it is "important to understand that conditioning lying is an essential component of patriarchal thinking for everyone" (p. 42). This is particularly relevant to the maternity system because reports of feeling coerced, lied to, and misinformed are rife in the obstetric violence literature (Jenkinson et al., 2017; Keedle et al., 2024). As bell hooks (2017) claims, "there can be no love without justice" (p. 19), but, as I argue in the next sections, with respect to maternity care, there can be no justice without love.

Relational midwifery thinking

A few years ago, Mavis Kirkham and I wrote a paper (Newnham & Kirkham, 2019), based on our individual ethnographic work, outlining the *problem* of autonomy as the basis for ethical care in midwifery practice. In this paper, we critiqued the principle of autonomy from a care ethics perspective, determining it an abstract and rhetorical concept which can obscure all manner of unethical practice (such as coercion), and therefore a poor cornerstone on which to hinge *informed consent* processes. Further work led by Kate Buchanan has identified the similarities between care ethics and midwifery philosophies (Buchanan et al., 2022). We continue interrogating the problem of autonomy, identifying that unless factors of power, oppression, and discrimination are openly recognised, the principle of autonomy does not function because it is based on the assumption that both parties are equally free and independent (Newnham & Buchanan, forthcoming). The delineation of autonomy as an abstract bioethical principle, and the problems associated with this, is not just a theoretical endeavour. It is an important point of departure for any discussion about how we are to address increasing violence within maternity systems, and what this might mean for ethical midwifery practice.

Ruddick's thesis on maternal thinking as providing grounds for a politics of peace identifies that oppressive and violent institutions and structures rely on abstracted language and concepts. Hyper-rational and abstracted terminologies such as "collateral damage" and "clean bombs" in militarist thinking are able to conceal what, in context, may involve "unspeakable human suffering" (Cohn, 1987, as cited in Ruddick, 1990, p. 146). Such terminology is purposefully used by such systems. They obscure the unique existence and unnecessary death of war victims, who as well as being *collateral damage* were also individual people with meaningful lives. Such abstractions enable violence, while contextualisation (understanding the human context) challenges violent behaviours, and in doing so, also confronts the structure of oppressive systems. And for these same reasons, adherence to *autonomy* as an abstract principle, without attention to power dynamics, can enable abusive or controlling behaviours, whereas care ethics, which requires attention to context and particularity, makes it much harder (if not impossible) to explain away violence of any kind.

If we take this argument to its conclusion, autonomy, as a principle of bioethics, appears to be unhelpful in the pursuit of bodily self-determination, even though at first glance, this seems to be what the autonomy principle is supposed to uphold. The right to determine what happens to your body, particularly when it comes to pregnancy and birth, is seen as an inalienable right, and underpins the reproductive justice framework (Ross & Solinger, 2017). In that case, what is needed is a different ethical cornerstone that can support maternity healthcare practitioners to fully realise bodily self-determination in the women they are caring for. What has been suggested is that *relationality* (or the process of relationship) could provide an alternative ethical cornerstone. The contextualising of ethical practice within *relationship* takes bodily self-determination from the abstract to the concrete and would therefore make it much harder for unethical, abusive, and disrespectful care practices to be carried out. In addition, it will help to redress moral distress (Foster et al., 2022, 2023, 2024) by aligning the practitioner's ethical allegiance to the woman/birthing person rather than the amorphous (abstract) institution (Buchanan et al., 2023; Chadwick, 2018; Feeley, 2023; MacLellan, 2014; Newnham & Kirkham, 2019; van der Waal & Nistelrooij, 2022).

These ideas are further developed in a paper outlining the unique position of midwifery as the (only) profession that participates in embodied practice to support the physiology of birth, and which has a long history of experiential and expert knowledge that both engages with technology and resists it (van der Waal et al., 2024). We termed this *somatophilic techne* (breaking this down to the root meanings of the words, *somato* refers to *the body*, *philia* to *affectionate love*, and *techne* to a form of knowledge combined of *art and skill*). This is a way of *thinking with the body*, of developing knowledge and practice (over centuries) with a positive affection and regard for the birthing body that capably holds the delicate balance between technology use (all forms, including pinards, robozo, abortion pills, and caesarean) and reproductive justice. We framed this unique combination of attributes as *relational midwifery thinking*, after Ruddick's *maternal thinking* (Ruddick, 1990; van der Waal et al., 2024; van Nistelrooij, 2022).

Following Ruddick, we identified for *relational midwifery thinking* the aims of "preservation of people and their capacity for pregnancy," "(un)becoming *motherandchild*," and "relations that support reproduction and reproductive freedom" (van der Waal et al., 2024, p. 21).

The aims of midwifery thinking, inherently relational, enable the material conditions which foster hooks' six elements of love. Whereas fragmented, time-poor, policy-bound systems of care foster abstracted and detached conditions which enable, if we follow Ruddick's logic, oppressive and violent beliefs and practices. In the next section, I discuss the importance of attention, and then link this to the idea of a *politics of love*, thereby making the case for love as necessary to justice.

Attentive love

Ruddick's focus on preservative love highlights the need for attentiveness in caring relationships (Bourgault, 2016; Ruddick, 1990), describing attention as "at once an act of knowing and an act of love" (Ruddick, 1990, p. 122). Attention (*knowing* the person, their context, and their needs and desires) and *love* (the will to extend oneself for the purpose of nurturing another's flourishing) are integral to relationality and an "important resource" of loving relationships (hooks, 2017, p. 163). The giving of attention enables one to be in the generous position of placing complete trust in the other. Central to Ruddick's interpretation of attention (or attentiveness) is a willingness to embrace difference, rather than looking for the shared comfort of similarities. If similarities are comforting, easy, and palatable, then being confronted with *otherness*, with unfamiliar ideas, thoughts, or experiences, requires us to sit with some discomfort. However, ultimately, by paying *attention* in this way, as an act of knowing and an act of love, it becomes possible to "let otherness be" (Ruddick, 1990, p. 122). That is, attentive love acknowledges the context, circumstances, aspirations, and desires of the other, and not only understands that these do not need to be the same as our own but encourages their pursuit.

Once we recognise this form of attention as central to a loving practice, it allows us to take a position of information sharing, guidance, and suggestion, but does not allow for persuasion or coercion in any way. This concept of attention allows for love and distance, of connection, of seeing oneself reflected in the other, as well as the ability to make space for their difference. Examples of this kind of practice abound in midwifery; however, most recently, it has been adeptly described in Claire Feeley's work on responsive midwifery (Feeley, 2023). In talking about their practice of supporting women who make birth choices outside of recommended guidance, midwives described high degrees of tension and risk to their professional autonomy or their employment. However, they were able to stand strong in their support for the astonishingly simple reason that they assumed "women had reasons for their decisions" (Feeley, 2023, p. 54). While holding this position of advocacy, midwives described experiencing pressure from others (colleagues, managers, doctors) to coerce women into decisions that fit the institution. This pressure to coerce is evidence of the *abstract violence* apparent within systems of care that cannot seem to acknowledge the absolute right of bodily self-determination; despite (or perhaps because of) autonomy being a cornerstone of bioethics and the foundation for *informed consent*. Such systems of care fail to comprehend this very basic concept, so perspicuously articulated by the midwives in Feeley's (2023) study: that birthing people have *reasons for their decisions*.

Midwives, generally, tend to support this process of collaborative decision making (Feeley, 2023). By open and transparent sharing of information, and working towards problem solving together, midwives can "widen women's choices" (Feeley, 2023, p. 55). Transparent, attentive, non-coercive sharing of knowledge that considers a person's context (their *reasons for decisions*) effectively reduces the power of the clinician, and increases the power held by the birthing person (Buchanan et al., 2023). This shift in power dynamic is a necessary condition for the possibility of bodily self-determination in maternity care.

Essential to all of this, of course, is first of all *to listen*. hooks (2017, p. 157) calls listening the "first responsibility of love," not only because it lets us hear the other's voice, but it also calls us to listen to our inner selves (whether this is thought of as intuition, or experiential knowledge, or conscience). For Ruddick (1990), listening, especially to voices who are traditionally silenced, distorted, or censored, is itself an act of resistance. Perhaps what is most crucial now is that midwives really listen to (collect and prioritise) our own knowledge and use our own (silenced) voices to "name the nameless so it can be thought" (Lorde, 1985 as cited in Ruddick, 1990, p. 40); to counter paternalistic, oppressive, patriarchal, and colonising discourses in maternity care. This means, researching areas that are important to women, birthing people, and midwifery practice, continuing the salutogenic discourse of childbirth, passing on experiential knowledge and practice expertise, and creating alternative systems of care that are external to obstetric models.

The politics of love: love as justice

As identified in the first sections of the chapter, part of the problem is that love and care are not prioritised in late capitalist economic systems. Drawing on the work of Erich Fromm and Martin Luther King, who were explicit in the *politicisation of love*, hooks identifies that "loving practice is not aimed at simply giving an individual greater life satisfaction; it is extolled as the primary way we end domination and oppression" (hooks, 2017, p. 76).

If one accepts the care ethics premise of human interdependence – that dependency is not unidirectional from carer to the one cared for, but that we are all dependent on each other (Newnham & Kirkham, 2019); this leads us to questions of need, privilege, and justice, and therefore underscores the political nature of care (Tronto, 2020). While "the neoliberal market does not, indeed cannot, value personal engagement, emotional connection, commitment, empathy or attentiveness, unless contracted for financial rewards" (Chatzidakis et al., 2020, p. 73), in actuality, we are all in need of all of these in order to flourish. Providing care with attention to particularity is therefore a key form of resistance to oppressive systems that rely on abstraction. Abstraction enables dehumanisation, and it is through the mechanism of abstraction (of bioethical principles, of policy-driven care, of fragmented institutional systems) that obstetric violence is enabled.

Following on from the points above, it can be argued that relational midwifery care that truly *lets otherness be* through loving attentiveness provides the necessary foundation to actualise bodily self-determination. However, it goes further than simple decision-making; these factors are central to human flourishing. To philosopher Simone Weil (Weil, 2024), consent is the central point of justice, because the conditions for true consent require equity. Where equity is not present, or where power relationships are not transparent, she argues, the need to obtain consent is diminished, or may not be acknowledged at all. This is relevant to the current status of maternity care systems, where *rhetorical autonomy* allows for coerced consent, ignoring the *reasons behind decisions*, particularly if they do not align with care provider recommendations (Feeley, 2023; Newnham & Kirkham, 2019), and without a transparent acknowledgement of the wielding of obstetric power and surveillance that occurs under the illusion of an autonomous consent process (Newnham, 2014).

Mimi Niles (2021) describes the work of midwifery in institutions as doing *kairos care* (which is relational and attentive) in *chronos time* (which is rigid, concerned with surveillance and control) within a tautological system that both defines and measures what is valued. What is valued are defined metrics, outputs, efficiency, which rarely incorporate the worth of human experience, an integral part of kairos care. In my own previous work, I have discussed the *paradox of the institution* (Newnham et al., 2018), which explains the mechanisms whereby *too much too soon* (Miller et al., 2016) occurs in maternity hospitals. This paradox identifies the way in which biomedicine, as a dominant paradigm, constructs medical practices as safe (e.g., induction, epidural analgesia), and others as risky (e.g., undisturbed birth, use of water immersion). Within this paradox, *institutional momentum* does not allow enough time to support birth physiology, but is in fact driven by an intervention ideology to surveil and speed up labour processes. There is a focus on keeping birthing women moving through the system to keep them safe from institutional systemic issues such as bed block, or from *long* labours, but which often (paradoxically) has the opposite effect of introducing risk (Shah, 2017). However, these institutional risks are not addressed or in fact noticed, due to the influence of the paradox. Within this system, while midwives can be placed in the role of normal birth *guardians*, they often do not, in actuality, have the time, the power, or the required trust in their knowledge by others, to practice in a way that really supports birth physiology. The lack of attention in maternity institutions to the knowledge systems and values of those working within it must now be seen as a form of epistemic injustice, that is, the ongoing suppression of midwifery knowledge (and midwives' practice) by its subjugation in relation to medical knowledge (and practice) (Allen, 2017; Newnham, 2014).

Careful loving attentiveness requires material conditions that can support adequate freedom over time and space (Weil, 1956, as cited in Bourgault, 2016). Institutions that are hurried, which operate at a pace where people are unable to "engage thoughtfully and creatively" (Bourgault, 2016, p. 77) undermine the capacity to listen, and therefore to truly pay attention. And thus, Weil places into a political context, if these conditions are not possible, then justice is not possible.

Love as humanisation: the way forward

Midwifery has a leading role in the work towards global reproductive justice, which it can achieve through a focus on relational midwifery thinking, somatophilic techne (art and skill developed in relationship with the body), and loving attentiveness. This will not only provide direct resistance to oppressive and dehumanising systems but also pave the way for reimagining an ethic of care for maternity systems.

The gathering of the Humanizing Birth Conference in Fortaleza, Brazil, in 2000, came up with the following definition (Umenai et al., 2001):

'Humanization'

A process of communication and caring between people leading to self-transformation and an understanding of the fundamental spirit of life and a sense of compassion for and unity with:

1 the Universe, the spirit and nature;
2 other people in the family, the community, the country and global society; and
3 other people in future, as well as past generations.

Humanization is an important means of encouraging and empowering individuals and groups to move towards the development of a sustainable society and the enjoyment of a fulfilling life.

Humanization can be applied to any aspect of care, including childbirth, the terminally ill, the elderly, the disabled, the poor, health and disease, education, the environment, economics, politics and culture.

This definition, with its reference to self-transformation, compassion, and interdependency, can clearly be linked to love: the practice of it; as well as the understanding of love as politics and love as justice. Humanising birth, then, is a justice project that has at its heart, a political loving practice that could be termed *loving praxis*, which does not stop at offering loving attention to individuals but understands it to be a form of resistance to oppressive dehumanising forces, and as fostering sustainability, community, and solidarity (Chatzidakis et al., 2020, p. 82). Loving praxis is an acknowledgement of the unique role that individual care and attention plays within the broader socio-political-economic systems that consistently deprioritise the behaviours and practices required to achieve these aims.

hooks (2017) explains how current dominant patriarchal, capitalist, and colonising patterns of thinking together form a *culture of domination*, characterised by oppression, control, and marginalisation; a culture that glorifies death rather than valuing life; a culture that dehumanises. This is echoed in Ruddick's (1990) discussion about the cultural privileging of war and violence. Just as maternal thinking creates space for a politics of peace, so midwifery thinking creates space for humanising birth. The focus on death (destruction), rather than life, inspires constant fear, of uncertainty, of loss of control, of death itself. It narrows and diminishes our experience. When this death-worship is challenged, when peace and justice are foregrounded, when a *love ethic* is embraced, chances can be taken, death becomes part of living, and we can live life to the full (hooks, 2017). This willingness to surrender, to be vulnerable, to face the possibility of one's own death, is at the heart of being able to freely relinquish one's own power in order to acknowledge the other's humanity; it is the crux of *letting otherness be* (hooks, 2017; Ruddick, 1990; Weil, 2024).

For midwives, the presence of love is also in the dedication to the role, so often described as a calling, a passion, a vocation. hooks (2017) cites Rainer Maria Rilke, who asserts that love has been misunderstood as only being about pleasure or play, but, he says: "there is nothing happier than work, and love, just because it is the extreme happiness, can be nothing else but work" (p. 183). So, we have come full circle in this chapter, relating the importance of love to the carrying out of midwifery work. Love is work, and midwifery work that encompasses loving praxis is necessary to achieve justice. Understanding this will take us one step closer to the goal of humanising birth.

References

Allen, A. (2017). Power/knowledge/resistance: Foucault and epistemic injustice. In I.J. Kidd., J. Medina., & G. Pohlhaus Jr. (Eds.) *The Routledge handbook of epistemic injustice* (pp. 187–194). Routledge.

Bourgault, S. (2016). Attentive listening and care in a neoliberal era: Weilian insights for hurried times. *Ethics & Politics/Etica e Politica, 18*(3). http://www2.units.it/etica/2016_3/BOURGAULT.pdf

Buchanan, K., Geraghty, S., Whitehead, L., & Newnham, E. (2023). Woman-centred ethics: A feminist participatory action research. *Midwifery, 117,* 103577. https://doi.org/10.1016/j.midw.2022.103577

Buchanan, K., Newnham, E., Ireson, D., Davison, C., & Bayes, S. (2022). Does midwifery-led care demonstrate care ethics: A template analysis. *Nursing Ethics, 29*(1), 245–257. https://doi.org/10.1177/09697330211008638

Chadwick, R. (2018). *Bodies that birth: Vitalizing birth politics.* Routledge.

Chatzidakis, A., Hakim, J., Littler, J., Rottenberg, C., & Segal, L. (The Care Collective) (2020). *The care manifesto: The politics of interdependence.* Verso.

Davis, D. A. (2019). Obstetric racism: The racial politics of pregnancy, labor, and birthing. *Medical Anthropology, 38*(7), 560–573. https://doi.org/10.1080/01459740.2018.1549389

Feeley, C. (2023). *Supporting physiological birth choices in midwifery practice: The role of workplace culture, politics and ethics.* Routledge.

Fleszar, L. G., Bryant, A. S., Johnson, C. O., Blacker, B. F., Aravkin, A., Baumann, M., Dwyer-Lindgren, L., Kelly, Y. O., Maass, K., Zheng, P., & Roth, G. A. (2023). Trends in state-level maternal mortality by racial and ethnic group in the United States. *JAMA, 330*(1), 52–61. https://doi.org/10.1001/jama.2023.9043

Foster, M. W., McKellar, L., Fleet, J. A., & Sweet, L. (2023). Moral distress in midwifery practice: A Delphi study. *Women and Birth: Journal of the Australian College of Midwives, 36*(5), e544–e555. https://doi.org/10.1016/j.wombi.2023.04.005

Foster, W., McKellar, L., Fleet, J. A., Creedy, D., & Sweet, L. (2024). The barometer of moral distress in midwifery: A pilot study. *Women and Birth: Journal of the Australian College of Midwives, 37*(3), 101592. https://doi.org/10.1016/j.wombi.2024.101592

Foster, W., McKellar, L., Fleet, J. A., & Sweet, L. (2022). Exploring moral distress in Australian midwifery practice. *Women and Birth: Journal of the Australian College of Midwives, 35*(4), 349–359. https://doi.org/10.1016/j.wombi.2021.09.006

hooks, b. (2017). *All about love: New visions.* Harper Collins.

Jenkinson, B., Kruske, S., & Kildea, S. (2017). The experiences of women, midwives and obstetricians when women decline recommended maternity care: A feminist thematic analysis. *Midwifery, 52,* 1–10. https://doi.org/10.1016/j.midw.2017.05.006

Keedle, H., Keedle, W., & Dahlen, H. G. (2024). Dehumanized, violated, and powerless: An Australian survey of women's experiences of obstetric violence in the past 5 years. *Violence Against Women, 30*(9), 2320–2344. https://doi.org/10.1177/10778012221140138

MacLellan, J. (2014). Claiming an ethic of care for midwifery. *Nursing Ethics, 21*(7), 803–811. https://doi.org/10.1177/0969733014534878

Mayra, K., Sandall, J., Matthews, Z., & Padmadas, S. S. (2022). Breaking the silence about obstetric violence: Body mapping women's narratives of respect, disrespect and abuse during childbirth in Bihar, India. *BMC Pregnancy and Childbirth, 22*(1), 318. https://doi.org/10.1186/s12884-022-04503-7

Miller, S., Abalos, E., Chamillard, M., Ciapponi, A., Colaci, D., Comandé, D., Diaz, V., Geller, S., Hanson, C., Langer, A., Manuelli, V., Millar, K., Morhason-Bello, I., Castro, C. P., Pileggi, V. N., Robinson, N., Skaer, M., Souza, J. P., Vogel, J. P., & Althabe, F. (2016). Beyond too little, too late and too much, too soon: A pathway towards evidence-based, respectful maternity care worldwide. *Lancet, 388*(10056), 2176–2192. https://doi.org/10.1016/S0140-6736(16)31472-6

Newnham, E. (2014). Birth control: Power/knowledge in the politics of birth. *Health Sociology Review, 23*(3), 254–268. https://doi.org/10.1080/14461242.2014.110 81978

Newnham, E., & Buchanan, K. (Forthcoming). Care ethics and midwifery. In I. van Nistelrooij, R. van der Waal, & V. Mitchell (Eds.), *Reproductive justice: Care ethics and beyond.* Peeters Publishers.

Newnham, E., & Kirkham, M. (2019). Beyond autonomy: Care ethics for midwifery and the humanization of birth. *Nursing Ethics, 26*(7-8), 2147–2157. https://doi.org/10.1177/0969733018819119

Newnham, E., McKellar, L., & Pincombe, J. (2018). *Towards the humanisation of birth. A study of epidural analgesia & hospital birth culture.* Palgrave Macmillan.

Niles, P. M., Vedam, S., Witkoski Stimpfel, A., & Squires, A. (2021). Kairos care in a Chronos world: Midwifery care as model of resistance and accountability in public health settings. *Birth, 48*(4), 480–492. https://doi.org/10.1111/birt.12565

Ross, L., & Solinger, R. (2017). *Reproductive justice: An introduction* (Vol. 1). Univ of California Press.

Ruddick, S. (1990). *Maternal thinking: Towards a politics of peace.* The Women's Press.

Sackett, D. L., Rosenberg, W. M., Gray, J. A., Haynes, R. B., & Richardson, W. S. (1996). Evidence based medicine: What it is and what it isn't. *BMJ (Clinical research ed.), 312*(7023), 71–72. https://doi.org/10.1136/bmj.312.7023.71

Sadler, M., Santos, M. J., Ruiz-Berdún, D., Rojas, G. L., Skoko, E., Gillen, P., & Clausen, J. A. (2016). Moving beyond disrespect and abuse: Addressing the structural dimensions of obstetric violence. *Reproductive Health Matters, 24*(47), 47–55. https://doi.org/10.1016/j.rhm.2016.04.002

Shah, N. (2017). *System Complexity and the Challenge of Too Much Medicine.* Keynote address. American Congress of Obstetricians and Gynecologists Annual Meeting. https://www.ariadnelabs.org/resources/articles/keynote-to-american-ob-gyns-c-section-rates-linked-to-hospital-complexities/

Thomas, K. (2024). *Listen to mums: Ending the postcode lottery on perinatal care: A report by the all-party parliamentary group on birth trauma.* https://www.theo-clarke.org.uk/sites/www.theo-clarke.org.uk/files/2024-05/Birth%20Trauma%20Inquiry%20Report%20for%20Publication_May13_2024.pdf

Tronto, J. (2020). *Moral boundaries: A political argument for an ethic of care.* Routledge.

Umenai, T., Wagner, M., Page, L. A., Faundes, A., Rattner, D., Dias, M. A., Tyrrell, M. A., Hotimsky, S., Haneda, K., Onuki, D., Mori, T., Sadamori, T., Fujiwara, M., & Kikuchi, S. (2001). Conference agreement on the definition of humanization and humanized care. *International Journal of Gynaecology and Obstetrics: The Official Organ of the International Federation of Gynaecology and Obstetrics, 75*(Suppl 1), S3–S4.

van der Waal, R., Mitchell, V., van Nistelrooij, I., & Bozalek, V. (2021). Obstetric violence within students' rite of passage: The reproduction of the obstetric subject and its racialised (m)other. *Agenda, 35*(3), 36–53. https://doi.org/10.1080/10130950.2021.1958553

van der Waal, R., & van Nistelrooij, I. (2022). Reimagining relationality for reproductive care: Understanding obstetric violence as "separation". *Nursing Ethics*, *29*(5), 1186–1197. https://doi.org/10.1177/09697330211051000

van der Waal, R., van Nistelrooij, I., Fox, D., & Newnham, E. (2024). Somatophilic rationality for reproductive justice: On technology, biological materialism, and midwifery. *Technophany, A Journal for Philosophy and Technology*, *2*(1), 1–32. https://doi.org/10.54195/technophany.13801

van Nistelrooij, I. (2022). *Humanizing birth from a care ethics perspective*. Keynote lecture at the Critical Midwifery Studies Summer School, Hosted by the University of Humanistic Studies. https://www.criticalmidwiferystudies.com/school

Watson, K., White, C., Hall, H., & Hewitt, A. (2021). Women's experiences of birth trauma: A scoping review. *Women and Birth: Journal of the Australian College of Midwives*, *34*(5), 417–424. https://doi.org/10.1016/j.wombi.2020.09.016

Weil, S. (2024). Are we fighting for justice? In D.K. Levy, & M. Barabas. (Eds., Trans.) *Simone Weil: Basic writings* (pp. 169–180). Routledge.

World Health Organization. (2014). *The prevention and elimination of disrespect and abuse during facility-based childbirth*. https://iris.who.int/bitstream/handle/10665/134588/WHO_RHR_14.23_eng.pdf

PART II
Love in practice

4

LOVE AS TOUCH

Claire Nutt

Introduction

The Roman poet and philosopher Lucretius wrote that "The paved highway of belief through touch leads straightest into the human heart and the precincts of the mind" (Trevelyan, 1920). Lucretius's words tell us that direct sensory experiences through touch have a powerful and immediate impact on human emotions and thoughts. The powerful impact of touch within midwifery practice will be explored in this chapter but perhaps the best place to start is with definitions.

Touch can be defined as an action, "to bring a bodily part into contact with, especially so as to perceive through the tactile sense: handle or feel gently usually with the intent to understand or appreciate" (Merriam-Webster online, 2024). This is an interesting explanation considering this chapter's focus on touch as a connecting expression of love. Facilitating an important presence and interaction that connects us with the world, touch enables us to feel around environments, navigating emotive connections. As one of the five core senses, touch provides an avenue of non-verbal presence for both giver and receiver. Although a gesture of touch can be unconscious and simple, the perception of it can be both complex and rewarding. In this respect, it is important to consider how touch is experienced maternally, neonatally, and from the perspective of the midwife. Simple adaptations to tactile routines can strengthen a sense of love within pregnancy, birth, and new parenthood. Considering the landscape of love within midwifery, this chapter seeks to define the foundation and action of touch and its key role within maternity care.

Traditionally embedded within midwifery culture, touch provides a vital toolkit within maternity care. Worldwide, as a soothing exploration and

DOI: 10.4324/9781032645780-7

reassurance, touch is used as both assessment and support. Seventeenth-century English midwives are recorded to have massaged women in labour with oil of lilies. The Japanese term for midwife is *samba, woman who massages*. For the Navajo (a native American people), the midwife is known as *the woman who holds*. In many South American midwifery cultures, including Yucatán and Zapotec communities, massage of the abdomen complements midwifery assessments. Additionally, pre-pregnancy deep uterine massage given by elders and midwives promotes reproductive health. In Jamaica, a midwife may rub a woman's abdomen with *toona* leaves and olive oil (Ananda, 2004). From abdominal palpation, a reassuring hand hold in labour, to the personal intimacy of vaginal examinations; how touch is approached by midwives and women impacts how caregiving is experienced.

The anatomy and physiology of touch

Tactile connection is perceived physically and psychologically. When touch occurs, varying afferent mechanoreceptors within the skin are activated, sensing pressure, temperature, proprioception, vibration, and stretch. In response, these receptors send signals to the cerebral sensory cortex of the brain, where areas vary in size to reflect the body area they respond to. These signals facilitate a complex sensation that blends sensory depth impact, texture and warmth, vigour of movement, and memory and context, ensuring that interpretations of a touch sensation are holistically intertwined (Hsiao & Gomez-Ramirez, 2011). What seems initially a simple stimulation is subjectively interpreted with great depth.

A positive aspect of this sensitive response to the context of touch is that due to varying touch response speeds of neurons, a slower response can promote calm and relaxation. An example is the activation of slow-responding C Tactile (CT) unmyelinated peripheral afferent fibres that respond specifically to stroking, particularly on areas like the forearm or back. This creates a pleasurable experience by triggering the slower paced *rest and digest* of the parasympathetic system, reducing heart and breathing rates (Pawling et al., 2017). Essentially, through the inhibition of an amygdala-based stress response and neurological activation of the rewarding effects of safety signals, this slower *feeling* overrides the stress response system.

More than this, stimulus is responded to with a complex blend of context, memory, and even sight and smell, to construct a physiological response that ripples throughout our being via the neuroendocrine pathways. This sensitive network results in a complex creation of serotonin and dopamine reward systems, oxytocic floods, and endorphin rich reactions, promoting a sense of relaxation and wellbeing (Bahrami et al., 2017; Field et al., 2009). Interestingly, this is a response similarly created by the holistic perception of emotion, safety, and warmth that is empathically stimulated in love (Brown, 2021).

Touch in pregnancy has a positive influence on fetal anatomy and wellbeing. From mid-pregnancy onwards melatonin, the hormone responsible for circadian rhythms promotes an ongoing chain reaction that includes fetal growth and laying down of fetal adipose tissue and stimulates growth of the fetal adrenals (Torres-Farfan et al., 2008). From the third trimester, maternal melatonin levels peak, in turn triggering more pronounced fetal-circadian adrenal responses and as a result, increased oestriol. Oestriol works in close synergy with oxytocin; therefore, there is an association between sleep, close social interactions, and a sense of wellbeing (Bates & Herzog, 2020). This hormonal "sisterhood" may be supported by encouraging partners to offer a massage each evening, when women are at the peak point of daily melatonin, with a vision not only to nurture sleep cycles but also build the hormonal foundation for physiological birth rhythms. The value of loving touch from carers and from partners is referred to throughout this chapter.

The complex messaging of hormones, connection, and feelings outlined above is influenced by the kind of touch that is made, the approach, the time, and how touch is responded to. This relies on intimate neuroendocrine stimulation and somatics that are deeply personal. Just as there are nuances of pain, emotion, and pleasure, as physical and psychological expressions, the way that touch is given has a powerful influence and its perception is subjective. The emotional context of touch is intrinsically intertwined with neuroendocrine complexities.

Touch and oxytocin

Oxytocin is a neurotransmitter produced within the hypothalamus, well recognised as the *love hormone* according to its effect on positive social interaction and wellbeing. Oxytocin is the keynote speaker that connects touch, love, and birth (Uvnäs-Moberg et al., 2014). Physiologically, McGlone et al. (2014) found that the aforementioned slow stroking stimulation of CT fibres promotes social bonding by connecting responses from the amygdala and hypothalamus, increasing the production of oxytocin, endorphins, and serotonin. These hormones encourage reciprocal empathy and salutogenesis through the action of reassuring touch (McNabb et al., 2006; Uvnäs-Moberg et al., 2014).

Montagu's seminal work: *Touching* (1986) and Uvnäs-Moberg's research (2011, 2013) consider the interwoven biological influences and psychosocial effects of touch and oxytocin. For example, animal studies found that *gentling* (stroking) increased health and courage and found that handling showed the most effect on *emotionality*. With increasing reports that people's experiences of isolation and stress are associated with anxiety, more research is needed that includes human responses to touch. However, the long-term psychosocial impact of oxytocin, stimulated by touch as a demonstration of loving attachment, adds a valuable dimension to the act of touch and massage in pregnancy and birth. Physical touch can enhance psychological relaxation, promoting soothing biochemical responses and distracting from stressful external factors. Massage is often provided in a private environment congruent to quiet contemplation, providing focused connections between a woman, partner, and their unborn child (Field, 2010; Lindgren et al., 2014). Interestingly, those that engage in meaningful touch and massage perinatally are more likely to use nurturing touch with their infants, continuing this oxytocin rich cycle (Field et al., 2008).

Touch is "fundamental to the human experience" (Durkin et al., 2021, p. 4). As a subjective human experience, touch is culturally influenced. Globally, there are significant variances of touch within cultural contexts that influence its meaning. Touching is diversely expected within human interaction across societies; cultural norms, and personal preferences shape how touch is perceived and expressed. Examples may be the welcoming handshake in the United Kingdom, the forehead-to-forehead breath exchange of the Hawaiian *honi*, or the frequency of touch in warm Mediterranean conversations to emphasise emotion. Touch connects communities.

Contrastingly, considering the inhibitors of loving touch in hospital environments within midwifery culture particularly, Ananda (2004) notes that medicalisation and obstetric intervention may be reducing touch in birth. Verny (1986) stated that the presence of technology in the labour room "is inversely proportional to the amount of human contact between staff and patient" (p. 41). The impact of excess technological dependence in childbearing must be thoughtfully considered and counterbalanced with contact (Ananda, 2004). As Uvnäs-Moberg (2013) recognised within her work on oxytocin, whilst caring relationships are intrinsically oxytocic, disconnected ward routines and techno-heavy tasks potentially eliminate opportunity for oxytocin-rich human connection.

Thankfully, there are ways to promote loving touch in all aspects of maternity care. Midwifery work has conscious and unconscious touch embedded within it. A midwife colleague shared with me that she habitually welcomes a woman and her partner to a birthing space with a warm handshake, encouraging rapport and quick connection, providing a great example of introducing conscious touch. Similarly, considering an abdominal palpation assessment, a woman can be invited to hold their abdomen first, gently wonder at the position and movements of her baby, and then the midwife begins to hold a focused abdominal touch for a second or two. By the midwife and woman being together, before abdominal palpation assessment begins in a gentle but conscious way, the parasympathetic system for the woman and potentially her baby is instigated, and a moment of physical connection begins that can be deeply effective.

To provide true unconditional regard, physical contact needs to be centred around personalised care. Whilst touch techniques can improve mental health by strengthening trusted relationships between midwives and families, this needs to be navigated with vigilance, respect, and shared understanding. Considering the therapeutic relationship between midwives and women, respecting emotional safety is imperative. We each bring a history of touch experiences that may evoke loving memories, but also those more fearful, potentially instigating threat or mistrust. Being conscious of how a physical approach can be perceived manipulatively, even violently, is vital to ensure tenderness is conveyed instead. Attitude, awareness, and intention of the touch-giver ensures touch has a loving focus whilst protecting the recipient's sense of feeling in control. This forms a foundation for trauma preventative and compassionate care.

Touch preferences can change from moment to moment, especially in labour. When consented and mutually adapted, it can be a very effective way to communicate, even in the most turbulent, challenging, and busy environment. In fact, one could argue this is exactly when mindful touch is most needed. Demonstrating care through touch, often alongside language, can foster tenderness within caregiving. This is particularly important given the cultural diversity and migratory nature of our populations which may mean that there are considerable language barriers. However, this highlights the crucial aspect of consent for touching, particularly for women who have experienced trauma and abuse, and are seeking sanctuary; not everyone wants to be touched. Yes, touch transcends verbal communication, but mutual agreement must still be mindfully sought for touch to be positively experienced. Loving touch in midwifery must complement other avenues of love such as words, time, and a woman-centred approach.

Massage as loving touch

Massage is considered an extension of touch, and widely used by women, partners, and midwives for birth (Redshaw & Heikkila, 2010). Massage may "convey concern, security, closeness and encouragement" with positive psychosocial impact (Chang et al., 2002, p. 72). Reflecting on the therapeutic encounter of massage, it is reported that recipients feel enjoyment whilst receiving massage and find the human, therapeutic approach both engaging and empowering; after receiving massage, participants report sleeping better (Smith et al., 2009). Others have found that by improving emotional wellbeing, massage promoted a heightened sense of *self-awareness* (Bahrami et al., 2017; Billhult & Maatta, 2009; Chang et al., 2002).

Massage utilises holds, strokes, and kneading movements to achieve rest, relaxation, and release (Field et al., 2008). The benefits of massage are associated with improved vagal activity and circulation, reduced heart rate, lowered blood-pressure, and reduced cortisol interestingly, for *giver* as well as receiver (McGowan, 2022). In Hawaii, the traditional massage *Lomilomi* is known as *the loving hands*; this approach to massage is not purely physical technique, but a two-way interaction involving the focused intention of both participants. The way that touch is given, the intention and emotion behind it, enhances the love, care, and compassion that is received. This feels reminiscent of midwives demonstrating compassionate care, such as through promoting a reciprocal approach to pregnancy and birth by encouraging birth partners to provide touch-focused support. For example, in Hawaii, some midwives teach partners massage as part of their antenatal care, to utilise in labour, both promoting neuroendocrine responses and empowering birth partners' own sense of calm, belonging, and participation.

Calm

Key themes reported when massage was used for labour and birth are that massage can reduce anxiety, provide comfort from labour, and promote a feeling of togetherness for both women and partners. Pregnancy, birth, and new parenthood present a natural stress that may for some be experienced as deep emotional challenge and strain.

Detrimental biological and psychosocial factors triggered by perinatal stress impact on the baby through the crucial, formative phase of pregnancy and onwards throughout childhood and adolescence, in turn influencing a cyclical detriment on their own parenting experience. Antenatal anxiety has been found to be a significant predictor of antenatal and subsequent postnatal depression with common association between the two (Bedaso et al., 2021). However, introducing soothing touch, such as massage in the perinatal period, can calm in times of stress (Eckstein et al., 2020).

Interventions such as massage reduce antenatal anxiety by addressing symptoms such as poor sleep, worry, and physical tensions. The Touch Institute, led by key researcher Tiffany Field, provides seminal research that finds massage reduces anxiety by preventing an increase in catecholamines (Field et al., 2008). Many massage group participants reported *less depressed mood, feeling better*, and *lower stress levels*. Partners also reported *lower maternal stress levels* and *greater labour progression*. Billhult and Maatta (2009) also explored the use of touch for anxiety, concluding that experientially massage was beneficial for recipients both in respect of *being relaxed in body and mind* and of *receiving unconditional attention*. Further assessment of neonatal outcomes and postnatal depression by Field (2014) also found positive results regarding reduced stress (through measured cortisol reductions) and improved connections with partners (in this case giving the massage) when massage was facilitated.

Comfort

In the experience of pain, it is instinctive to want to *rub it better*. Pain is essentially subjective and complex. A holistic response to soothing touch may include distraction, feeling supported and neurological stimulation combined. In labour particularly, touch becomes an essential tool for supporters to provide comfort. A Canadian study of massage for labour in a hospital environment explored pain scores alongside experiences of massage therapy (Adams et al., 2010). They reported that "overall pain, emotional-wellbeing, relaxation, and the ability to sleep" is improved by massage (p. 4). In addition, women reported improved satisfaction with their birthing experience, shorter labour times for some, and those who planned an epidural found they waited longer to request pain relief (Adams et al., 2010; Lai et al., 2021; Nutt, 2016a).

A combined opioidergic, analgesic activity of endorphins stimulated by touch, with an oxytocin boosting sense of shared experience; therefore a reduction of fear improves experiences of pain. Touch-techniques such as holding, stroking, and acupressure alleviate discomfort and promote physiological and neuroendocrine processes of birth, whilst simultaneously assisting the woman's ability to cope (Smith et al., 2009; Tiran & Chummun, 2004).

More robust research and exploration of women's perceptions are needed to fully explore what massage in labour really means to women and partners; however, a repeated theme in several studies, including Field et al. (2008) and McNabb et al. (2006), was the inclusion of partners. Touch techniques can be easily taught to partners in pregnancy in preparation for birth, empowering relationships between couples, improving shared experiences of maternity care and as a result, supporting a family-centred and loving approach to parenthood (Ditzen et al., 2007).

Connection

A connection can be defined as the relationship, or link, between one thing (in this context a person) and another. This could be the physical link of direct touch, shared time, and experience, or a sense of belonging. The term *haptic* means an extension of touch that comes "through the total experience of living and acting" (Montagu, 1986, p. 17). In a world where technology often influences and even dominates our interactions, a mindful introduction of haptics ignites a physical connection to our everyday technology such as mobile phones (the vibration you feel when a message arrives stimulates a dopamine response), although human touch remains the most potent and essential means of connection. Rubin (1963) said that in "intense personal stress, situations in which one feels isolated and vulnerable, there seems to be no other modality comparable to touch in the immediacy of effective response" (p. 828). Disconnected relationships enhance feelings of isolation and loneliness, and symptoms of depression and anxiety can exacerbate poor relationships. Therefore, a shared experience of loving touch strengthens relationships, and is key to family health. Touch as connection shows empathy, support, and intimacy. Two of Field's studies (2008; 2009) teach the *significant others* to give massage throughout pregnancy. They found that giving massage proved most effective when women received massage from partners, promoting a relaxed response more quickly than if given by a stranger.

McNabb et al. (2006) and Kimber et al. (2008) use a programme of massage as preparation and practice for labour in late pregnancy, supported by studies that find long-term benefits for both women and partners when massage is shared. When a course of massage is practised by a couple prior to a *stressful event*, there is a direct protective effect on stress-related neurobiological systems, "as a possible underlying mechanism of health beneficial effects of positive couple interaction" (Ditzen et al., 2007, p. 566). Therefore, this reduction in stress ripples like a wave through the recipient, touch-giver, and the midwife as observer.

A somatic approach focuses on the impact of sympathetic responses to touch, alongside the psychosocial connection of a dynamically therapeutic relationship, promoting partner inclusion whilst encouraging psychological relaxation and self-confidence (Billhult & Maatta, 2009). A midwife can promote touching between a woman and partner, physically and psychosocially, particularly in labour as part of a family-centred approach. Additionally, it is noted by Field (2014) that those couples, who use massage together in pregnancy and labour, were more likely to massage their infants postnatally.

Touch and the neonate

Touch is the parent of our eyes, ears, nose, and mouth. It is the sense which became differentiated into the others, a fact that seems to be recognised in the age-old evaluation of touch as the mother of the senses.

(Montagu, 1986, p. 3)

The very word *attachment* evokes a sense of being together, connected through touch. The first seeds of attachment for a newborn to their mother is a vital element of midwifery care and stimulates a pathway to love for new families (Shoghi et al., 2018). Skin-to-skin, for example, provides a meaningful and practical experience of touch. Beyond thermoregulation, this first touch conveys a safe, sensory, and deeper connection for babies (Ferber et al., 2008).

Touch is fundamental to family connections, as a mindful and multi-sensual activity for both parents giving, and infant receiving, alike. In addition to skin-to-skin, touch is received by babies through abdominal massage in pregnancy, during breastfeeding, and through neonatal massage which stimulates biological growth and neural development, calming parasympathetic responses and prompting full sensory reactions to the world around them (Hardin et al., 2021). There is a growing body of evidence that supports touch for newborns throughout their development and lifespan (Kahalon et al., 2022; Trivedi, 2015).

Playing a crucial role in early neonatal health and social development, touch strongly influences a baby's emotional safety; a tactile conversation that tenderly contributes to building a loving family environment (Cascio et al., 2019).

Moreover, many studies on massage for premature and newborn babies reveal how regular touch and massage promote growth by stimulating appetite, calming an anxious baby, and ensuring a sense of security (Field, 2010; Underdown, 2009).

Positive touch for babies can be simply incorporated into everyday activities, such as focused changing, feeding, and carrying. Touch is naturally incorporated in breastfeeding. Focused massage time can be developed into routines such as bathing or before sleep, suiting family life rhythms. Essentially by being held, by feeling safe, cortisol responses are reduced. By holding their baby, parents themselves can feel empowered, soothed, and confident in their own and their baby's emotional growth (Yanviv et al., 2021).

Touch encourages a sense of togetherness

Touch, as a form of love connection, joins up families (Nutt, 2016b). Positive touch reassures a baby that they are not alone, tells them that all is safe in the world, that they are cared for, and their emotional needs are being met (Nutt, 2020). Connection is the key to effective newborn massage; through presence of mind, reduced distraction, and collaboration, attachment begins. Author Winnicott (1965) seminally stated that a baby in utero is not considered as being alone. Bergner et al. (2008) highlight that a dyadic intervention, a two-way approach that clearly unites mother and child, is fundamental given how maternal wellbeing evokes significant alterations in neurobiological layers of the baby. This togetherness reduces cortisol, soothes, and improves appetite by promoting feeding responses when close.

Another interesting aspect regarding touch which fosters love, friendship, and support, relates to the *togetherness* of midwives, and touch between each other, that in turn may promote more loving care in clinical practice. There are stories of midwives massaging each other on shift. Not all midwives may want to give or receive massage per se, but a shared experience of touch or even observing it, can stimulate wellbeing responses. Essentially, touch-centred midwifery care, care given with a loving touch, can also stimulate wellbeing responses for midwives. Providing touch within the workplace can prompt reciprocal benefits and may ripple positively through teams; a mindful approach and connection with colleagues may vicariously influence touch within caregiving when experienced warmly. Relationship-centred working supports relationship-centred care. We need fellow midwives and clinicians to have their hands on our backs, whether that is real or perceived.

Ultimately, connection improved by loving physical interactions brings togetherness within the mother–baby relationship, the partnership of parents, the family, and midwifery colleagues. From establishing trust and connection during pregnancy to providing comfort and guidance during labour and postpartum, throughout caregiving, loving touch is a powerful tool that tenderises experiences. Through loving compassionate touch, the physical, emotional, and spiritual heart of midwifery is held.

References

Adams, R., White, B., & Beckett, C. (2010). The effects of massage therapy on pain management in the acute care setting. *International Journal of Therapeutic Massage and Bodywork*, *3*(1), 4–11.

Ananda, K. M. (2004). The primal touch of birth: Midwives, Mother's & Massage. *Midwifery Today Magazine*, 70.

Bahrami, T., Rejeh, N., Heravi-Karimooi, M., Vaismoradi, M., Tadrisi, S. D., & Sieloff, C. (2017). Effect of aromatherapy massage on anxiety, depression, and physiologic parameters in older patients with the acute coronary syndrome: A randomized clinical trial. *International Journal of Nursing Practice*, *23*(6), 1–10. https://doi.org/10.1111/ijn.12601

Bates, K., & Herzog, E. D. (2020). Maternal-fetal circadian communication during pregnancy. *Frontiers in Endocrinology*, *11*, 198. https://doi.org/10.3389/fendo.2020.00198

Bedaso, A., Dams, J., Peng, W., & Sibbritt, D. (2021). The association between social support and antenatal depressive and anxiety symptoms among Australian women *BMC Pregnancy and Childbirth*, *21*, 708. https://doi.org/10.1186/s12884-021-04188-4

Bergner, S., Monk, C., & Werner, E. (2008). Dyadic intervention during pregnancy? Treating pregnant women and possibly reaching the future baby. *Infant Mental Health Journal*, *29*, 399–419.

Billhult, A., & Maatta, S. (2009). Light pressure massage for patients with severe anxiety. *Complementary Therapies in Clinical Practice*, *15*, 96–101.

Brown, B. (2021). *Atlas of the heart*. Penguin House.

Cascio, C.J., Moore, D., & McGlone, F. (2019). Social touch and human development. Developmental Cognitive Neuroscience, *35*, 5–11.

Chang, M., Wang, S., & Chen, C. (2002). Effects of massage on pain and anxiety during labour: A randomised controlled trial in Taiwan. *Journal of Advanced Nursing*, *38*(1), 68–73.

Ditzen, B., Neumann, I. D., Bodenmann, G., von Dawans, B., Turner, R. A., Ehlert, U., & Heinrichs, M. (2007). Effects of different kinds of couple interaction on cortisol and heart rate responses to stress in women. *Psychoneuroendocrinology*, *32*(5), 565–574. https://doi.org/10.1016/j.psyneuen.2007.03.011

Durkin, J., Jackson, D., & Usher, K. (2021). The expression and receipt of compassion through touch in a health setting: A qualitative study. *Journal of Advanced Nursing*, *77*(4), 1980–1991. https://doi.org/10.1111/jan.14766

Eckstein, M., Mamaev, I., Ditzen, B., & Sailer, U. (2020). Calming effects of touch in human, animal, and robotic interaction—Scientific state-of-the-art and technical advances. *Frontiers in Psychiatry*, *11*. https://doi.org/10.3389/fpsyt.2020.555058

Ferber, S. G., Feldman, R., & Makhoul, I. R. (2008). The development of maternal touch across the first year of life. *Early Human Development*, *84*(6), 363–370. https://doi.org/10.1016/j.earlhumdev.2007.09.019

Field, T. (2010). Touch for socioemotional and physical well-being: A review. *Developmental Review*, *30*(4), 367–383.

Field, T. (2014). *Touch* (2nd ed.). MIT Press.

Field, T., Deeds, O., Diego, M., Hernandez-Reif, M., Gauler, A., Sullivan, S., Wilson, D., & Nearing, G. (2009). Benefits of combining massage therapy with group interpersonal psychotherapy in prenatally depressed women. *Journal of Bodywork and Movement Therapies*, *13*(4), 297–303. https://doi.org/10.1016/j.jbmt.2008.10.002

Field, T., Figueiredo, B., Hernandez-Reif, M., Diego, M., Deeds, O., & Ascencio, A. (2008). Massage therapy reduces pain in pregnant women, alleviates prenatal depression in both parents and improves their relationships. *Journal of Bodywork and Movement Therapies*, *12*(2), 146–150. https://doi.org/10.1016/j.jbmt.2007.06.003

Hardin, J. S., Jones, N. A., Mize, K. D., & Platt, M. (2021). Affectionate touch in the context of breastfeeding and maternal depression influences infant neurodevelopmental and temperamental substrates. *Neuropsychobiology*, *80*(2), 158–175. https://doi.org/10.1159/000511604

Hsiao, S., & Gomez-Ramirez, M. (2011). Chapter 7. Touch. In: J.A. Gottfried. (Ed.) *Neurobiology of Sensation and Reward*. CRC Press/Taylor & Francis. https://www.ncbi.nlm.nih.gov/books/NBK92803/

Kahalon, R., Preis, H., & Benyamini, Y. (2022). Mother-infant contact after birth can reduce postpartum post-traumatic stress symptoms through a reduction in birth-related fear and guilt. *Journal of Psychosomatic Research*, *154*, 110716. https://doi.org/10.1016/j.jpsychores.2022.110716

Kimber, L., McNabb, M., Mc Court, C., (2008). Massage or music for pain relief in labour: A pilot randomised placebo-controlled trial. *European Journal of Pain*, *12*(8), 961–969.

Lai, C. Y., Wong, M. K. W., Tong, W. H., Chu, S. Y., Lau, K. Y., Tan, A. M. L., Hui, L. L., Lao, T. T. H., & Leung, T. Y. (2021). Effectiveness of a childbirth massage programme for labour pain relief in nulliparous pregnant women at term: A randomised controlled trial. *Hong Kong medical journal = Xianggang yi xue za zhi*, *27*(6), 405–412. https://doi.org/10.12809/hkmj208629

Lindgren, L., Jacobsson, M., & Lämås, K. (2014). Touch massage, a rewarding experience. *Journal of Holistic Nursing*, *32*(4), 261–268.

McGlone, F., Wessberg, J., & Olausson, H. (2014). Discriminative and affective touch: Sensing and feeling. *Neuron*, *82*(4), 737–755. https://doi.org/10.1016/j.neuron.2014.05.001

McGowan, S. (2022). The effects of pregnancy massage on mother and baby. *Journal of Health Visiting*, *10*(11). https://doi.org/10.12968/johv.2022.10.11.464

McNabb, M. T., Kimber, L., Haines, A., & McCourt, C. (2006). Does regular massage from late pregnancy to birth decrease maternal pain perception during labour and birth? A feasibility study to investigate a programme of massage, controlled breathing and visualization, from 36 weeks of pregnancy until birth. *Complementary Therapies in Clinical Practice*, *12*(3), 222–231. https://doi.org/10.1016/j.ctcp.2005.12.006

Merriam-Webster. (2024). *Online dictionary*. https://www.merriam-webster.com/dictionary/touch

Montagu, A. (1986). *Touching; The human significance of the skin* (3rd ed.). Harper & Row.

Nutt, C. (2016a). Discussing the evidence: Massage as a positive experience. *MIDIRS Midwifery Digest*, *26*(2), 195–199.

Nutt, C. (2016b). How can the use of massage in labour improve the experience of birth for women? *MIDIRS Midwifery Digest*, *26*(2), 64–73.

Nutt, C. (2020). Calm, comfort and connection for family well being. *The Practicing Midwife, 23*(4), 1–2.

Pawling, R., Cannon, P. R., McGlone, F. P., & Walker, S. C. (2017). C-tactile afferent stimulating touch carries a positive affective value. *PLoS One, 12*(3), e0173457. https://doi.org/10.1371/journal.pone.0173457

Redshaw, M., & Heikkila, K. (2010). *Delivered with care, a national survey of women's experience of maternity care*. University of Oxford.

Rubin, R. (1963). Maternal touch. *Nursing Outlook, 11*, 828–829.

Shoghi, M., Sohrabi, S., & Rasouli, M. (2018). The effects of massage by mothers on mother-infant attachment. *Alternative Therapies in Health and Medicine, 24*(3), 34–39.

Smith, J., Sullivan, J., & Baxter, D., (2009). The culture of massage therapy: Valued elements and the role of comfort, contact, connection and caring. *Complementary Therapies in Medicine, 17*, 181–189.

Tiran, D., & Chummun, H. (2004). Complementary therapies to reduce physiological stress in pregnancy. *Complementary Therapies in Nursing & Midwifery, 10*(3), 162–167. https://doi.org/10.1016/j.ctnm.2004.03.006

Torres-Farfan, C., Richter, G., & Germain, A. (2008). Melatonin and pregnancy in the human. *Reproductive Toxicology, 25*, 291–303.

Trevelyan, R.C. (1920). *Translations from Lucretius (Book V)*. George, Allen and Unwin Ltd. The Project Gutenberg eBook of Translations from Lucretius, by R. C. Trevelyan.

Trivedi, D. (2015). Cochrane review summary: Massage for promoting mental and physical health in typically developing infants under the age of six months. *Primary Health Care Research & Development, 16*(1), 3–4.

Underdown, A. (2009). The power of touch – Exploring infant massage. In: J. Barlow & P. Swanberg, (Eds). *Keeping the baby in mind- infant mental health practice*. Routledge.

Uvnäs-Moberg, K. (2011). *The oxytocin factor; Tapping the hormone of calm, love and healing*. Pinter & Martin.

Uvnäs-Moberg, K. (2013). *The hormone of closeness; The role of oxytocin in relationships*. Pinter and Martin.

Uvnäs-Moberg, K., Handlin, L., & Petersson, M. (2014). Self-soothing behaviors with particular reference to oxytocin release induced by non-noxious sensory stimulation. *Frontiers in Psychology, 5*, 1529. https://doi.org/10.3389/fpsyg.2014.01529

Verny, T. R. (1986). The psycho-technology of pregnancy and labor. *Pre- and Perinatal Psychology Journal 1*(1). 31–49.

Winnicott, D. (1965). *The Maturational processes and the facilitating environment: Studies in the theory of emotional development*. International Universities Press.

Yanviv, A., Salomon, R., Waidergoren, S., & Feldman, R. (2021). Synchronous caregiving from birth to adulthood tunes humans' social brain. Proceedings of the National Academy of Sciences, 118(14). article id:e2012900118.

5

LOVE AS ACTIONS

Indie Luna

Introduction

In considering the expression of love through action in midwifery, much of what can be discussed is painted with one of two brushstrokes. The first encompasses the role of the midwife as a clinician providing care, and the ways a midwife chooses to approach this are unique to each particular relationship developed with those under her care, and, of course, responsive to changing circumstances. A large part of this involves touch (see also Chapter 4), a hand holding another; and as in any profession where physical contact forms a part of the expected interactions, love plays a key role in guiding the appropriate behaviour of those involved, particularly those leading the relationship, which in most cases is the midwife. This love is manifested as respect, trust, even, at times, affection. Loving midwifery acts also encompass advocacy, providing information as well as enhancing midwifery knowledge and clinical competency.

The second is the sometimes less acknowledged, but nevertheless important, pivotal place midwives hold in the movement to challenge the socio-political inequalities faced by so many. Here, love is demonstrated through the midwife's desire to create an environment in which those in their care can thrive. And this goes further than the oxytocin-enriching low lighting and quiet music during a birth, and instead focuses on the wider context, on social justice, women's rights, and sexual and reproductive empowerment, considering the structural phenomenon of injustice and addressing it accordingly.

For either of these to achieve any success, it requires choices to be made by midwives, both as individuals but also as part of a wider collective, and it is in making these that the guiding influence of love can be demonstrated. Midwives are required to move beyond the conceptualisation of love as a passive

DOI: 10.4324/9781032645780-8

emotion, and instead embrace the potential that it can act as a dynamic force, removed from sentimentality, and instead moving towards encompassing a wide range of actions and attitudes that reflect a deep commitment to the well-being and dignity of every individual, and then intentionally integrating this into both clinical practice and social activism.

Respect, compassion, empathy, affection, commitment, trust, protectiveness, empowerment, amity, and any number of other contributory emotions, each of these stands alone in their own right, and can certainly be effectively argued to be quite different from a singular concept of love. But when these are brought together as a cohesive entity embedded within the midwife–mother dyad, or between midwifery colleagues, that is where they exist instead as demonstrative elements of love. In midwifery, love becomes the embodiment of the collective experience, it becomes the action of expressing each element, moving fluidly between them, and often expressing more than one in tandem. Stories of midwives expressing love as an action are present everywhere, from the highlands of Ethiopia to the forest of the Democratic Republic of Congo, and several are included throughout this chapter.

Acts of love in clinical practice

Grounded in philosophy and morality, in research and reality, the evidence shows there is huge potential in acts of love to have impact not only on quality of care, but on the lived experience of those both giving it and receiving it (Fitzgerald, 2005).

The relationships formed between midwives and those in their care, by the very nature of the context within which these meetings happen, occur at a time of heightened emotions often of huge complexity. Recognising and responding to this is the first act of love a midwife can take. In so doing, the midwife is required to have an empathetic understanding of the vulnerability created, and the potential for the resultant power imbalance to render the chance of true informed consent impossible (Henderson, 2003). Given that informed consent is the foundational cornerstone of clinical care (Cook, 2016), and the first and most important tenet that a midwife establishes as she offers it, demonstrating love in this context requires the midwife to act in such a way that overcomes this power imbalance to place another at the centre of the conversation. Advocating for women, upholding their sovereign autonomy over their body in order to facilitate their ability to make decisions about their health and care (whether or not the midwife ultimately agrees with the choices made) is the starting point.

From there, there is unity between midwife and mother. It is possible to recognise the creation of a new entity, the *syncytium* that Vouzavali et al. (2011) talk of in their research, into the role love plays in critical care nursing. This is the *we* of the midwife and woman together, connected in a symbiotic relationship, in addition to the two existing as independent individuals.

This becomes apparent when considering even the casual conversations that might happen between midwives passing in a labour ward corridor, and one asks the other how it's going, with the latter replying "We're getting there. We'll have this baby soon." For this moment in time, for the length of the created relationship, the boundaries of the identity of the midwife have broadened to include the woman in her care, with their experiences becoming hers; their joys in finding a fetal heartbeat for the first time, their excitement in the first contractions, their frustrations at the challenges of navigating the healthcare systems. Love here becomes the midwife's choice to invest in this relationship, to support and encourage, to empower, to act in such a way that their knowledge and skill is used for the betterment of the experience of another. Unusually perhaps for love, in the context of midwifery, it both results in relationships that bring together individuals that may otherwise occupy very different social locations in a unique moment of interconnectedness, whilst also recognising the transient nature of this moment. It isn't a love built on an extended experience of intimacy and connection; it can be a relatively fleeting shared instant that has considerable impact despite that.

Because of the brief nature of this unique form of love, each interaction becomes even more important, which in turn can act as a driving force behind a midwife's desire to ensure their own clinical competency. If a midwife recognises that providing high-quality clinical care, given that is what contributes in no small part to a positive experience for women and their families, is an act of love, then that can justify why a midwife may be willing to sacrifice their own time. Whether this is to pursue continuing professional development opportunities, or to stay on beyond the end of their shift to observe an unusual case, or to give up a weekend to enrol on a clinical skills course, these sacrifices are considered worth it. Choosing to enhance one's own clinical competency beyond the required minimum is a reflection of the element of love that means a midwife moves beyond selflessness, and instead understands the necessity for self-sacrifice if it leads to the betterment of the experience of another, committing to another's wellbeing and putting their needs beyond her own, even when it's difficult. This is the affective nature of love in midwifery, where it becomes a driving force encouraging one to seek out chances that allow the choice to act with love to become realised. Fitzgerald and Stan Van Hooft (2000) recognised this in nursing too and commented that the nurses most highly thought of were those that moved beyond the legalistic view of duty of care, and to love in the act of professional caring. Below is a story of a midwife in Ethiopia doing just this.

It isn't often that midwives in Ethiopia are given the opportunity to attend university and gain a bachelor's degree in addition to the college-level diploma that many practice with. When that chance does arise though, even when it means travelling far from home for months at a time over the course of years, to attend the lectures and classes put on by university staff during the holidays, they will do everything to find a way to make it possible. Often this means working days and nights for weeks to raise the funds, selling precious zebu cattle or roasting coffee or baking injera to make up any shortfall, as well as taking small loans from friends and family. Education is sacrosanct, because the midwives know that the knowledge they have is, quite literally, the difference between life and death for those in their care. Engider is one such woman who is now the proud holder of a degree. She left behind her families, her young children, her home for three months over keremt (the rains) each year for five years, travelling for days by bus over the mountains far to the east of the country to make it happen.

So many of the skills learnt by midwives, whether these are those gained through going above and beyond or otherwise, rely on physical contact, from palpating to feel the lie of an unborn baby, to the intimate examinations performed during a birth, to breastfeeding support, to a hug of congratulations, or of commiserations. Whatever the nature of this touch, it must always be performed with consent, with evidenced reason, with trust, and with privacy and dignity in mind. But love can also play a role, too. As in life, love here becomes acting in such a way that moves beyond the bare necessities, in small gestures of kindness that may be seemingly insignificant, but that make a tangible difference to the experience of those in the midwife's care. This can be anything from warming gel before a vaginal examination to holding their hand whilst sharing unexpected news. With the increased medical complexity of many pregnancies, and the need for more procedural management of these, as well as the increasing role of technology in healthcare, there is a risk that the human touch will be lost. Midwifery, as in healthcare more generally, has adapted to incorporate advances in medical knowledge and technology, but must also preserve the core values of empathy, advocacy, and compassion. Given love as touch has been discussed in Chapter 4, not much more needs to be said here, except to reiterate that each time a midwife reaches out to those in her care, how she chooses to do so provides a time and a space where love in action can be apparent. It is all too clear that, not only within the UK NHS, but in many other countries with health systems that are under-staffed and over-wrought, having enough time to love is becoming a vanishingly rare event, which is all the more reason to recognise that even the briefest of moments has the potential to provide a platform for acts of love.

Because of the intimacy inherent in pregnancy and birth, trust plays a fundamental role (O'Brien et al., 2021). In as much as those bringing new life into the world (be that the woman, her birth partner, or her wider family) must place their trust in their midwife, so too must the midwife trust those in her care. The decisions the midwife makes about recommendations for care are based not only on her own biophysical findings, but also on the information given to her. If this is inaccurate, or incomplete, there is a chance that the midwife's care choices are no longer appropriate, and may, in certain cases, even be unsafe, with the potential for a cascade of avoidable issues, the blame for all of which will sit at the feet of the midwife. Trust, then, becomes a fundamental reciprocal foundation stone on which the relationship must rest. Those under the care of the midwife trust her with their care, and in turn the midwife trusts them with her livelihood. As with many other sentiments such as empathy, compassion, or affection, acts of trust aren't necessarily synonymous with acts of love. But when taken as part of the wider context of the provision of midwifery care, it becomes a contributory element to love. The image of love as a diamond, described in Chapter 2, comes to mind here. Like a diamond, love has many different faces. Trust is one of those faces.

Whilst the majority of time as a midwife is spent caring for women, in a demonstration of love through action, there are other relationships to consider. Foremost amongst them are that of the midwife and the baby, and that of the midwife and her colleagues. The first of those, for reasons that probably don't need explaining, is far easier to imagine embracing. Handling a newborn with affection, carrying out any clinical checks with gentleness, and creating an environment of love doesn't always require a deviation from expected clinical standards, and can even, more often than not, be evidenced as the gold standard. For example, encouraging new parents to maintain skin-to-skin contact (with simple but research-based advice as to why this is beneficial) (Moore et al., 2016) or delaying disruptive checks that are not time sensitive (the easy example here is head circumference or weight, which does not need to be performed within the first minutes, or even hours, of a healthy baby's life) (Sharma, 2017) are two simple ways. Likewise, engaging in discussions around the environment of the room (things like not allowing bright lights and loud, sudden movements, to avoid startling the newborn) (Mercer et al., 2007), which may seem more like actions based in our biophysiological understanding of a neonate rather than anything else. But taking the time to understand each, to explain each, and to encourage each, even when it seems impossible under the circumstances of a busy labour ward, is both loving and brave. In the days and weeks following the birth, for the period of time that the newborns still fall under the care of the midwife, whether on a postnatal ward, a neonatal unit, or in the community, more opportunities to demonstrate love are likely to arise. From warming up a baby's heel to ensure that a newborn blood spot test is carried out as gently as possible, to helping new parents understand what normal neonatal behaviour is, in order to alleviate unnecessary stress in the family; a midwife's love for a newborn lends itself to creating an environment within which the new baby can thrive. The story below demonstrates a loving midwifery act.

A little over a year ago, in rural Cheha Woreda, Ethiopia, a young first-time mother, Woinshet, experienced eclamptic seizures. She was rushed into emergency surgery, and the subsequent caesarean section saved her life, and that of her son. For hours after the birth, though, she remained unconscious, with a newborn who needed feeding. Her midwife, Atsede, stepped in. With a baby of her own still nursing, and plenty of milk for both, there was never any question that she would feed her baby son too. For those moments that Atsede sat there, a woman able and willing to feed a baby, a midwife doing what was needed for those in her care, she embodied love in action.

A little more challenging, perhaps, than acting with love towards a sweet newborn, is doing so with an overworked, underappreciated colleague teetering on the edge of their own limits. It is possible that a supporting, loving work environment can be cultivated in midwifery, and whilst this seems a long way from the experiences of many at the moment (Capper et al., 2021; Gillen et al., 2004; Simpson et al., 2023; … the list of relevant research here could go on and on), if each midwife takes responsibility for their own actions, and reactions, and chooses to ground these in love, change would soon materialise. There are innumerable ways that midwives can act with love, from fostering atmospheres of open communication, where colleagues feel comfortable expressing thoughts and concerns, to listening actively and encouraging each other to share experiences and insights. Equally important is recognising the challenges that each may face in both their professional and personal lives, and showing empathy and offering support when needed, as well as understanding that every member of the team has different strengths and weaknesses. This allows individuals to approach situations with a mindset of cooperation rather than judgement. Collaboration, rather than division, must be emphasised within the healthcare team, with the contributions of all members, from the consultant obstetricians to the student midwives, the catering staff to the healthcare assistants, acknowledged and appreciated. If each is open to learning from another, valuing the unique expertise that everyone can offer, and fostering a collaborative culture of continuous learning by sharing knowledge and resources, the overall competence of the team increases.

Building a strong, cohesive foundation upon which a clinical service can lean doesn't mean relying on the occasional team-building yoga session, but instead strengthening relationships and fostering a sense of unity every day, every shift, through simple expressions of gratitude for a colleague's hard work and dedication, through celebrating achievements, however seemingly significant or otherwise, and through acknowledging the unique skill sets that each member brings to the team. Small gestures go a long way in fostering a positive environment. For new staff, either students who have just qualified or those moving in from another role, entering an already established culture can be intimidating, with complex hierarchical dynamics to consider. So, if each midwife chooses to offer either formal or informal mentorship to new colleagues, sharing their experiences to help navigate the role, and providing support during transition periods, either with practical guidance or just a listening ear, this will go a long way in providing a more welcoming, easily managed transition.

It is inevitable that conflict and disagreements will arise, such is the nature of a group of humans working together in an often high-stress environment, but addressing these with a constructive and compassionate approach, and seeking resolution through open dialogue leads to a much better understanding of each other's perspectives. Each midwife can make the choice to maintain a harmonious working environment, forgiving the mistakes and missteps of colleagues, moving forward with a focus on learning from these, rather than apportioning blame and encouraging gossip. To do so is to act with love, and by incorporating these principles into each midwife's daily interactions, their workplace culture can become supportive, compassionate, and built on a foundation of respect. Ultimately, a positive and loving work environment benefits not only the wellbeing of the staff, but also enhances the quality of care provided to women and their families.

Acts of love in social activism

As is widely recognised, the role of the midwife transcends just the provision of clinical care, encompassing a commitment towards fostering a just and equitable socio-political environment. At its very core, midwifery is about nurturing life, and whilst this manifests most often in guiding women and their families through a pregnancy and birth, there is also the pivotal role midwives play in embracing a broader perspective that acknowledges the impact of cultural, economic, political, and social factors on care, and a commitment towards dismantling barriers that hinder access to it. The multi-faceted challenges of social injustices often weave insidious threads into the healthcare systems, affecting marginalised communities disproportionately, resulting in a tangible cycle of poor outcomes. Issues such as racial disparities, lack of access to and awareness of services, and discriminatory politics that perpetuate inequality, sit at the heart of why. By providing care based on a philosophy of embracing acts of love, midwives contribute to a positive experience, with empowered women more likely to engage in proactive health practices, leading to better outcomes for both mother and child. This next story shows the positive impact midwives can make.

In Gurage Zone, Ethiopia, the gowza tribal system influences much of life, from marriage to skills learnt to the continuation of harmful traditional practices. Amongst the Funga, who are viewed in much the same way as the Dalit caste in Hindu India, often facing social exclusion and discrimination, female genital circumcision persists, even when many of the Gurage gowza have abandoned the custom. It takes great strength of character to stand against a centuries old tradition, but when midwives Selam and Aster attended the birth of a baby girl born into the Funga, they knew that their words in the first few hours and days of the child's life could change what would come next. Sitting with the baby's mother, Selam and Aster drew diagrams, explained clinical textbooks, shared their own stories, drank coffee together, reached out to hold her hand, arranged meetings with the Protestant priest and her in-laws, and were determined to approach the situation with gentleness, kindness, empathy, and love, rather than the judgement and dismissal the Funga were all too used to receiving. Both of the baby's parents agreed with a quiet but resolute certainty that their daughter would be spared cutting. Three years later, this woman returned to Selam and Aster for the birth of her second child, two years after that, the birth of her third, and another two years later, her fourth. Each time, these parents proudly spoke of their resistance to having their eldest daughter cut, despite overwhelming pressure from their families. Without Selam and Aster choosing love in a moment of heightened emotion, it is likely there would have been very different conversations between the midwives and the young Funga mother.

In considering how to challenge the present circumstances through advocating for change, love once again acts as a dynamic force, fostering determination in midwives to leverage their expertise in navigating complex landscapes to create an environment where everyone, regardless of their background, can experience comprehensive, compassionate healthcare with dignity and without fear of discrimination. Recognising the importance of cultural competence, actively engaging with diverse communities to bridge gaps in understanding and challenging the status quo that perpetuates discrimination and implicit bias, lay the groundwork for dismantling the systemic racism embedded in healthcare systems and reforming an inclusive and sensitive midwifery service. Standing up against social injustice is a multi-faceted endeavour. Midwives must: advocate for policies that support equitable representation and ensure that diverse voices are contributing towards shaping practice; confront economic inequalities that impact access to quality care; and challenge patriarchal norms and push for autonomy; and agency and work to create an environment where those accessing midwifery care are empowered to make informed choices about their bodies and health. Midwives can choose to participate in research investigating the impacts of social determinants on maternal health outcomes, and in so doing, this act of love becomes a catalyst for dismantling the structures that perpetuate discrimination. By contributing to developing an empirical evidence base to support recommendations, with a focus on fostering an environment that bridges the gap between privileged and disadvantaged communities, and recognising that access to comprehensive, compassionate maternal healthcare should not be a matter of luck but a human right, midwives play a pivotal role in bringing about social change. Contributing to community wellbeing also relies on the promotion of maternal and infant health education, through encouraging engagement in outreach programmes and initiatives, focusing on empowering women with knowledge, fostering a culture of informed decision-making, and proactive health management.

Making an active choice to engage in self-reflective practice, with an awareness and understanding of one's own biases, and through empathetic understanding, midwives can choose to connect with the wide-ranging experience of those in their care and recognise the intersectionality of their identities with unique challenges faced. When caring for those who have previously experienced poor outcomes because of incompetent care, for example, love provides the motivation to recognise the ways that women may carry the weight of their past experiences, and how this affects their expectations for, and experiences of, subsequent clinical care. This may mean enrolling in formalised ongoing professional development courses in birth trauma resolution or similar, or simply choosing to engage with the multitude of online learning opportunities that come with following the social media accounts of diverse and passionate clinicians and service users discussing these issues. Love fuels a commitment to continuous education and self-reflection, acknowledging that both handling the consequence of social injustice as well as looking towards dismantling these altogether requires an ongoing effort. Midwives must challenge biases within themselves, and within their profession, striving to provide care that is not only clinically competent but also culturally sensitive and inclusive.

In many societies, women face restrictions on their reproductive and sexual health choices, and often risk condemnation or even violence should they choose to ignore these. It is also in those same societies, despite decades or centuries of denunciation and censure from patriarchal authorities, that midwives consider it both a professional duty and moral obligation to work towards dismantling these oppressive structures. Ensuring autonomy and self-determination for women through their reproductive journey, as well as their lives more generally, and empowering women to make informed decisions about their bodies and families may be the rationale, but in talking to midwives in such situations, love is a perceptible driving force behind why many risk their own livelihoods, and lives, to protect the choices and rights of the women in their care. The sacrifice made by one midwife is described below.

In 2020, Akello, a passionate, devoted Alur midwife from Mahagi territory, Democratic Republic of Congo, was arrested and imprisoned, spending almost a year in jail whilst her community, her hospital, and her lawyers fought to have her released. Her crime was providing terminations to teenage girls who had fallen pregnant as a result of the sexual violence perpetrated by armed guerrilla groups during the ongoing conflict in the country. The Congo has very restrictive laws surrounding the provision of abortifacients, enforced by local police officers, who often act at the behest of the *big men* in the communities, many of whom view successful, outspoken women with distrust and anger. Aware of this, and understanding the inevitable consequences should she be caught, Akello chose to sacrifice her own freedom to care for the girls in her community. Her story ends happily, with her release and reinstatement as a midwife.

Midwives engaged in protesting social injustices must also navigate the delicate balance between professionalism and activism. Bound not only by national and international law, but also by the guidance of the governing bodies in whichever country they are practising, be that the Nursing and Midwifery Council in the United Kingdom, or the FDRE Ministry of Health in Ethiopia, midwives are not only individuals but also, simultaneously and inescapably, representatives of a wider profession. If a midwife were to participate in a protest that involves illegal actions, for example, it can jeopardise their professional standing, with significant consequences. Given this, decisions made, and actions taken by a midwife, must honour both elements of her identity, balancing advocacy with maintaining ethical and professional integrity. That said, midwives must often walk the finest line between prioritising the empowerment and care of women and adhering to potentially harmful, restrictive laws and cultural norms. And when love, which is so much harder to ignore than a sense of professional duty, is understood as the motivation for action, it becomes even more challenging. In some parts of the world, the impact of such actions can be dangerous and devastating as described below.

Binta, a Fulani midwife from Wurno, Sokoto State, Nigeria, was chased from her home, which was then set alight, after the council of local Islamic elders discovered she had been providing contraception and sex education to other women in this conservative, traditional community. No longer able to practise openly, and at risk of further danger, she fled to Abuja, where she found work as a midwife with WHARC (Women's Health and Action Research Centre). Her story, whilst rarely heard, is not unusual. Many will remember reading of Maryam Noorzad, a midwife at Dasht-e-Barchi maternity ward, who was murdered by Taliban gunmen for refusing to leave the side of a woman in labour.

Examples of acting with love to stand up for injustice, and the resultant fallout that midwives endure, need not be as extreme as the stories of Binta, or Maryam, or Akello. In the UK, especially recently, there has been a growing movement of midwives and associated birth professionals calling out the poor treatment of those who choose to stand up against an increasingly medicalised system, advocating for maternity care reform and questioning unnecessary interventions. Even when prioritising women-centred care, even when supported by the evidence base, if these actions are seen as questioning the status quo, a move that, historically, is not well accepted by established medical practices, midwives often face criticism, reproach, even ostracism. If anything, this goes to show both how powerful love can be, and how important it is to recognise that love as a motivation is worth fostering, as it provides the inspiration to stand up against injustice, even when it seems impossible.

Final words

Midwives have a choice to make. Each must decide whether to crumble under the weight of the myriad challenges facing the profession, whether to walk away, whether to rage and weep, or whether to love; to stand up for those in their care, for each other, for the endless possibilities that come with the seminal moments through which they walk; to accept that challenges and conflict are as inevitable in midwifery as they are in life; and to recognise that caring for the people on the edge of the night means that despite the heartache, the sadness, the disappointment, despite all of it, midwives can choose to care, to empower and advocate, to demand change, to lend the weight of their knowledge and experience and passion, and be with women, through the fear and the anticipation, through all of it, and to act with love.

References

Capper, T., Muurlink, O., & Williamson, M. (2021). Social culture and the bullying of midwifery students whilst on clinical placement: A qualitative descriptive exploration. *Nurse Education in Practice*, *52*, 103045. https://doi.org/10.1016/j.nepr.2021.103045

Cook, A. (2016). Midwifery perspectives: The consent process in the context on patient safety and medico-legal issues. *Journal of Patient Safety and Risk Management*, *22*(1–2), 22–29.

Fitzgerald, L. (2005). *Metaphysics of love as moral responsibility in nursing and midwifery*. Deakin University.

Fitzgerald, L., & van Hooft, S. (2000). A socratic dialogue on the question 'what is love in nursing? *Nursing Ethics*, *7*(6), 481–491. https://doi.org/10.1177/096973300000700604

Gillen, P., Sinclair, M., & Kernohan, G. (2004). A concept analysis of bullying in midwifery. *Evidence-Based Midwifery*, *2*(2), 46–51. https://link.gale.com/apps/doc/A167030950/AONE?u=anon~b19b3166&sid=googleScholar&xid=35c4b0bb

Henderson, S. (2003). Power imbalance between nurses and patients: A potential inhibitor of partnership in care. *Journal of Clinical Nursing*, *12*(4), 501–508. https://doi.org/10.1046/j.1365-2702.2003.00757.x

Mercer, J. S., Erickson-Owens, D. A., Graves, B., & Haley, M. M. (2007). Evidence-based practices for the fetal to newborn transition. *Journal of Midwifery & Women's Health*, *52*(3), 262–272. https://doi.org/10.1016/j.jmwh.2007.01.005

Moore, E. R., Bergman, N., Anderson, G. C., & Medley, N. (2016). Early skin-to-skin contact for mothers and their healthy newborn infants. *The Cochrane Database of Systematic Reviews*, *11*(11), CD003519. https://doi.org/10.1002/14651858.CD003519.pub4

O'Brien, D., Butler, M. M., & Casey, M. (2021). The importance of nurturing trusting relationships to embed shared decision-making during pregnancy and childbirth. *Midwifery, 98*, 102987. https://doi.org/10.1016/j.midw.2021.102987

Sharma, D. (2017). Golden hour of neonatal life: Need of the hour. *Maternal Health, Neonatology and Perinatology, 3*, 16. https://doi.org/10.1186/s40748-017-0057-x

Simpson, N., Wepa, D., Vernon, R., Briley, A., & Steen, M. (2023). Midwifery students' knowledge, understanding and experiences of workplace bullying, and violence: An integrative review. *International Journal of Nursing Studies Advances, 5*, 100144. https://doi.org/10.1016/j.ijnsa.2023.100144

Vouzavali, F. J., Papathanassoglou, E. D., Karanikola, M. N., Koutroubas, A., Patiraki, E. I., & Papadatou, D. (2011). 'The patient is my space': Hermeneutic investigation of the nurse-patient relationship in critical care. *Nursing in Critical Care, 16*(3), 140–151. https://doi.org/10.1111/j.1478-5153.2011.00447.x

6

LOVE AS WORDS

Anna Marsh

Introduction

Whilst words may feel like one of the simplest ways to demonstrate love, it is undeniable that they also hold a complex web of nuance and context. How something is said, who it is said by or in what situation it is used, can add to, alter, or turn upside down the simple meaning of a word or phrase. Within midwifery, we use words every day to communicate with women and our staff teams, but how often do we stop and think about how we use words and their power? The words and language midwives use not only impact those who they provide care to, but also with each other and the broader interdisciplinary team. Reports have highlighted that workplace bullying is rife within maternity services (Hunter et al., 2017; Kirkup, 2022), with a study citing it as a key reason why midwives leave the profession (Royal College of Midwives [RCM], 2016). Considering the current known shortages of midwives in the United Kingdom and in many other parts of the world, reducing bullying and improving how we communicate could be argued as a key solution to the ongoing midwifery staffing crisis. Our use of words and language is a significant factor in this. This chapter will explore the benefits of expressing love through words within midwifery, and what happens when we don't. It will also touch on the power of using a more loving language with women, colleagues, and with ourselves. It will then explore the potential future of words as we progress to an increasingly digital age.

DOI: 10.4324/9781032645780-9

Love as words with women

Without realising it, we are expressing love through our communication in our daily roles. It is known that building and nurturing a relationship with women is essential for high-quality care, and that it is a key part of the role of a midwife (Almorbaty et al., 2023). Using words and communicating in a meaningful, compassionate way is fundamental to building a relationship.

Whether written or verbal, perhaps one of the most basic elements of the role of a midwife is to communicate using words. Communication is central to high quality, safe maternity care (Kirkup, 2015; National Maternity Review Team, 2016; Ockenden, 2022) and essential for true informed consent and decision making (Stapleton et al., 2002). However, the words that midwives share with those they are providing care for around the world have great power to both create positive and negative impact. Midwives' have a critical role in providing appropriate information because they are the central point of contact with women throughout pregnancy, birth, and the postnatal period. The words and language they use throughout this time is key.

To some, the concept of midwives using *words with love* when talking to women may feel a bit alien at first. When considering examples of *words with love* within our personal lives, initially we think of more direct interactions like saying "I love you" in a romantic context. A study found that saying "I love you" to your romantic partner demonstrates a "commitment to future actions" (Ackerman et al., 2011, p. 1079). To apply the same sentiment to our professional practice, it could be argued that synonyms of "I love you" when used within a professional capacity could be "I'll see you for your next appointment in two weeks," "How do you feel about that?," or "Would you like a cup of tea?." This could even be extended to sharing evidence-based information, compassionate emotional support or just an appointment time or location update.

However, in our personal lives, we use words to show love in a range of other ways, not only by just saying "I love you." Considering how we speak to our partners, our families, our friends and even with our colleagues, communicating love is often far more indirect. Asking someone how they are, enquiring about family or sharing an inside joke may also be how we express love through words.

Communicating with love is not just about the words spoken, but how they are spoken. Healthcare professionals using a more positive or warm tone of voice has been found to improve service users' experiences and feelings about their care, as well as their perception of their own health and response to treatments (He et al., 2018; Weyant et al., 2017). On the other hand, when healthcare professionals use a more negative tone of voice with patients, it has been found to show lack of empathy or even lack of interest in their roles (Kee et al., 2018). When considering the repetition of some of the things midwives tell women in routine care, such as when discharging them from the postnatal ward or in antenatal appointments, tone of voice is something we need to be mindful of.

A study exploring the effects of healthcare professionals wearing masks on service users during the COVID-19 pandemic (Marler & Ditton, 2021) found that tone of voice was essential for communicating our own emotions, of which love could be included. Whilst this may seem less relevant post-COVID-19, this should still be considered, especially when caring for people with sensory disabilities, neurodiversities, or receiving care in an operating theatre where face masks are still worn.

The benefits of using words with love

Women are known to have a better birth experience if they feel listened to, and build a trusting relationship with their midwife and receive compassion (Karlström et al., 2015; Mannava et al., 2015; Ménage et al., 2017), which are all communication-based concepts. Considering this, using words and language lovingly when we speak with women clearly has the potential to directly influence their health and experience. As advocates and supporters of women during the childbearing journey, reducing their pain, easing their transition to motherhood, and empowering them through positive communication are fundamental to what midwives do.

There are significant benefits to using words with love with those we care for. Research has shown that the words that healthcare professionals use can have a directly positive psychological impact on patients, even to the extent of physical impact such as lowering their pain (Howick et al., 2018; Vranceanu et al., 2012). In the context of midwifery, the affirmations that we say such as "You are doing really well!" or "Keep going!" to women in labour are said with positive, perhaps even loving, intention to support them in their journey. Continuity of carer is a fundamental concept to improving communication between women and midwives. Key national reports have highlighted continuity of carer as essential for service users and their babies (National Maternity Review Team, 2016; Ockenden, 2022), with the key focus on the woman–midwife relationship achieved through continuity as a tool for improving outcomes (Sandall et al., 2016). Central to the woman–midwife relationship is the presence of trust (Mirzaee & Dehghan, 2020), with effective interaction found to be an essential element. Linking back to what we know about communicating with love, this trust can only be enhanced by love and a commitment to future actions. Such a commitment is made more possible through continuity of carer.

Whilst words and how we say them may be half of communication, listening is the essential other half that must not be ignored. Asking how a woman is, may be said lovingly, but without truly listening to the answer, it cannot be a caring, loving approach. Listening ensures that we are providing a woman-centred service, and is fundamental to compassionate care (Menage et al., 2020). With increasing demands on the midwifery workforce, short staffing and long to-do lists may make listening an easy thing to overlook, but taking the time to do this is essential when caring lovingly.

Using words without love

Whilst communication and the words we use may have powerful positive effects, we also know that they can negatively affect the women within our care. For example, using medicalised words has the power to increase the perceived severity and rareness of an illness (Young et al., 2008). The Re:Birth campaign (RCM, 2022) highlighted that commonly used medical terms such as *failure to progress* and *incompetent cervix* are received as demeaning to women, negatively impacting their experience. Whilst these may be part of routine maternity vocabulary, these phrases can cause harm and offence to women as the language suggests a fault or problem with their body or birthing ability. Such words are directly linked to birth trauma, an increasingly pertinent topic around the world (Watson et al., 2021). Whilst these may be routinely used phrases, it is unlikely that healthcare professionals are using them maliciously or with intent to offend. However, particularly to people using the service for the first time or without medical knowledge, like many of our service users, it is understandable how these terminologies may be perceived as lacking in love and how for some women they are harmful.

This may highlight a bigger problem than just clumsy, old-fashioned terminology. Considering that pregnancy and birth are largely a normal life event, the concept of *overdefinition* may come into play. Overdefinition, put simply, is where we create long complicated words for something that is ultimately a normal thing, and it is increasingly a problem in healthcare (Aronson, 2022). An example of this may be *Spontaneous Rupture of Membranes* for the very normal process of *waters breaking*. This label could make it sound like a complex medical condition, possibly even an abnormal one; the word *rupture* alone may sound quite dramatic! Overdefinition aligns with highly medicalised approaches to pregnancy and birth. Within maternity services today, language is under scrutiny and needs to be reviewed and updated. There is a line to be tread though, where language can be accurate and clear but not unnecessarily frightening and exclusive. The language should work for those women receiving low risk care based on a salutogenic model (Perez-Botella et al., 2015) and for those needing high risk care.

The words used within maternity services may also have the power to exclude the very people we are trying to reach. It may seem obvious that none of the impact of words can reach those within our care if we aren't speaking the same language, but it is essential to highlight this as an area we are continuously failing at. Within the UK, women facing a language barrier have significantly higher mortality and morbidity than native English speakers (Knight et al., 2023). Despite this, the use, documentation, and regulation of interpreters remains inconsistent across maternity services with many NHS Trusts delivering maternity services reporting significant issues with access and provision (MacLellan et al., 2024). In the UK interpreting provision is under review, but institutional use of these services is continually encouraged (NHS England, 2023).

Additionally, maternity services are traditionally designed for heterosexual women, often excluding those who do not identify as such. Misgendering (using incorrect gender pronouns) or heteronormative words can negatively affect the experience of service users, for example, those from the LGBTQ+ network (McCann et al., 2021). These areas for potential exclusion of service users highlight a significant area for improvement and opportunity to reduce inequalities to the people we care for. Communicating with love in these circumstances is about having an open and honest conversation, including asking service users how they would like to be addressed and if there are words or terms they would prefer us to use. For example, providing the opportunity at the first engagement with maternity services for the person to tell us their preferred pronouns.

Love as words with colleagues

As explored within Chapter 10, Love and Colleagues, the midwifery workforce is undeniably facing testing times across the world at present with increasing pressures on workload and stress. The words that we use when speaking with our colleagues are essential for promoting love and ensuring our own psychological safety and a culture of civility. It is known that workplace bullying and incivility is present within maternity services (Hunter et al., 2017; Kirkup, 2022). Despite this, research has shown that the more we receive caring, loving interactions from our colleagues, the more engaged we are and the better we perform (Barsade & O'Neill, 2014). Therefore, reviewing and improving how we communicate to colleagues, with a fundamental focus on love, may be essential for the future of our midwifery workforce. This will be explored in more detail in Chapter 10.

Using words with love amongst a team is everybody's responsibility; however, it is undeniable that leaders have a key role in creating a more positive culture. A study found that respectful, compassionate leadership directly correlated with a more positive culture within a ward (Papadopoulos et al., 2020). Compassionate leadership is a style highlighted by the RCM recently as fundamental and uses a loving, supportive approach, utilising the four elements of *Attending*, *Understanding*, *Empathising*, and *Helping* to improve workforce culture (RCM, 2021). To ensure a more loving maternity culture moving forward, this approach to leadership, especially with regard to the language we use, needs to be emulated by all, including everyone from student midwives to those in the most senior positions. As will be highlighted by Chapter 12, using and encouraging positive, loving language with our students will underpin their careers and improve the workplace cultures of the future.

Love as words with ourselves

A full exploration of love for ourselves can be found in Chapter 9 but it is worth exploring a little here with regards to words. Demonstrating love to yourself using words may sometimes feel uncomfortable and is rarely a routine part of our 21st century lives. However, research has shown that self-affirmations, or positive comments to ourselves, can improve wellbeing, decrease stress, and even make people more open to behaviour change (Cohen & Sherman, 2014). To put simply, if we make a conscious effort to be more positive and kinder to ourselves, there is significant potential for it to improve our lives and practice as midwives.

One practical way in which we can use words of love to improve our own wellbeing is through the use of mindfulness. Self-care is known to be essential to maintain wellbeing and resilience, and many find mindfulness a flexible, realistic tool to facilitate this within our day-to-day lives (Sist et al., 2022). Whilst there are a range of mindfulness courses and tools, they are all under-pinned with giving yourself time, space, and kindness. Speaking to ourselves with love throughout, mindfulness can nurture our relationship with ourselves and support our wellbeing in the long term (Solhaug et al., 2019).

Love as words, the future

In an increasingly digital era, consideration needs to move towards the future of words within maternity services. Communication around the world has evolved exponentially as the internet has become a routine part of our lives, and online words are slowly becoming just as loud, or arguably often louder, than the ones we say in a busy midwifery clinic. This presents a new opportunity to communicate with love and enhance the midwife–woman relationship of the future.

Is this an opportunity to improve care? From emojis to memes, from TikTok videos to viral dances, how people communicate and foster relationships, is now a multimedia phenomenon, and perhaps it's time that midwives got involved. Adapting our language to ensure it translates onto the internet, this could be a new opportunity to communicate with love to people we care for and reap the benefits for both midwives and women.

Social media is becoming a hub for pregnant women, often being referenced as a key place for information sharing and being part of a motherhood commu-nity (Baker & Yang, 2018; Morse & Brown, 2022a; Sanders & Crozier, 2018).

This suggests that social media is already becoming a supportive, perhaps even loving, space for childbearing women to build a community. Despite this, very few midwives engage with social media within our professional roles, leaving information sharing and discussion without professional support or guidance (Marsh et al., 2023a). Without our presence and with very limited research into the area, it is hard to know whether social media is proving a safe platform for discussion and support amongst pregnant people or a negative, even dangerous, environment.

Around the world, midwives are beginning to use social media more. In the USA, for example, social media is used more commonly by midwives where it is often used as a tool for advertising services (Marsh et al., 2023b). It is also being used to give a voice to women and to address common misconceptions, and to empower and improve their experiences (Marsh & Lowry, 2023). We are somewhat behind our US colleagues in the UK with social media rarely a routine part of our roles as midwives. However, often in response to the COVID-19 pandemic, local examples of midwives using social media are increasingly becoming visible. One example is the AskAMidwife service which was highlighted in the National Neonatal and Maternity review as a trailblazing innovation, using Facebook and Instagram as a way for clients to access a midwife (Marsh et al., 2024). Additionally, several examples of small *private* social media groups consisting of service users and midwives have demonstrated significant value to all (McCarthy et al., 2017; McCarthy et al., 2020; Morse & Brown, 2022b; Morse & Brown, 2023). More research is required to explore the effect of such services and the impact on the midwives and women involved, but this could demonstrate a new opportunity for midwives to communicate with women. Social media could be the new platform for midwives to communicate with love to build the woman–midwife relationship, empower them with information, and improve their experiences and outcomes.

Whilst using social media may seem a far cry from our more traditional midwifery practice, perhaps collaborating with experts in communication from the fields of media, communications, and marketing could be a way for midwives to navigate this relatively new online language.

Conclusion

Whilst using loving words and language within our roles as midwives may not be quite as obvious as within our personal lives, by empowering a woman with information, making a plan to see her again, or enquiring as to her wellbeing, we are demonstrating loving words on a daily basis. Using loving words with those within our care, our teams and ourselves underpins our core values as midwives and promotes wellbeing. However, there is significant potential to damage the experience of people using maternity service or reduce inclusivity if we use words without love.

As communication within the modern world continues to evolve in new and increasingly digital ways, how we utilise words as tools for providing care will grow. Considering the impact of communicating with love within a team to promote collaboration, or even with ourselves to promote resilience, using loving words more often may even be the solution to many of the current problems facing maternity services.

References

Ackerman, J. M., Griskevicius, V., & Li, N. P. (2011). Let's get serious: communicating commitment in romantic relationships. *Journal of Personality and Social Psychology*, *100*(6), 1079–1094. https://doi.org/10.1037/a0022412

Almorbaty, H., Ebert, L., Dowse, E., & Chan, S. W.-C. (2023). An integrative review of supportive relationships between child-bearing women and midwives. *Nursing Open*, *10*(3), 1327–1339. https://doi.org/10.1002/nop2.1447

Aronson, J. K. (2022). When I use a word .... Too much healthcare-overdefinition. *BMJ*, *378*, o2019. https://doi.org/10.1136/bmj.o2019

Baker, B., & Yang, I. (2018). Social media as social support in pregnancy and the postpartum. *Sexual & Reproductive Healthcare: Official Journal of the Swedish Association of Midwives*, 17, 31–34. https://doi.org/10.1016/j.srhc.2018.05.003

Barsade, S. G., & O'Neill, O. A. (2014). What's love got to do with it? A longitudinal study of the culture of companionate love and employee and client outcomes in a long-term care setting. *Administrative Science Quarterly*, *59*(4), 551–598. https://doi.org/10.1177/0001839214538636

Cohen, G. L., & Sherman, D. K. (2014). The psychology of change: Self-affirmation and social psychological intervention. *Annual Review of Psychology*, *65*, 333–371. https://doi.org/10.1146/annurev-psych-010213-115137

He, X., Sun, Q., & Stetler, C. (2018). Warm communication style strengthens expectations and increases perceived improvement. *Health Communication*, *33*(8), 939–945. https://doi.org/10.1080/10410236.2017.1322482

Howick, J., Moscrop, A., Mebius, A., Fanshawe, T. R., Lewith, G., Bishop, F. L., Mistiaen, P., Roberts, N. W., Dieninytė, E., Hu, X.-Y., Aveyard, P., & Onakpoya, I. J. (2018). Effects of empathic and positive communication in healthcare consultations: a systematic review and meta-analysis. *Journal of the Royal Society of Medicine*, *111*(7), 240–252. https://doi.org/10.1177/0141076818769477

Hunter, B., Henley, J., Fenwick, J., Sidebotham, M., & Pallant, J. (2017). *Work, Health and Emotional Lives of Midwives in the United Kingdon: The UK WHELM study*. https://pre.rcm.org.uk/media/2924/work-health-and-emotional-lives-of-midwives-in-the-united-kingdom-the-uk-whelm-study.pdf

Karlström, A., Nystedt, A., & Hildingsson, I. (2015). The meaning of a very positive birth experience: focus groups discussions with women. *BMC Pregnancy and Childbirth*, *15*(1), 251. https://doi.org/10.1186/s12884-015-0683-0

Kee, J. W. Y., Khoo, H. S., Lim, I., & Koh, M. Y. H. (2018). Communication skills in patient-doctor interactions: Learning from patient complaints. *Health Professions Education*, *4*(2), 97–106. https://doi.org/10.1016/j.hpe.2017.03.006

Kirkup, B. (2015). *The report of the morecambe bay investigation*. https://assets.publishing.service.gov.uk/government/uploads/system/uploads/attachment_data/file/408480/47487_MBI_Accessible_v0.1.pdf

Kirkup, B. (2022). *Reading the signals. Maternity and neonatal services in East Kent— The report of the independent investigation*. Department of Health and Social Care. https://www.gov.uk/government/publications/maternity-and-neonatal-services-in-east-kent-reading-the-signals-report

Knight, M., Bunch, K., Felker, A., Patel, P., Kotnis, R., Kenyon, S., 7 Kurinczuk, J.J. (Eds.) (2023) *Saving lives, improving mothers' care care – Lessons learned to inform maternity care from the UK and Ireland confidential enquiries into maternal deaths and morbidity 2019-21*. MBRRACE UK. https://www.npeu.ox.ac.uk/assets/downloads/mbrrace-uk/reports/maternal-report-2023/MBRRACE-UK_Maternal_Compiled_Report_2023.pdf

MacLellan, J., McNiven, A., & Kenyon, S. (2024). Provision of interpreting support for cross-cultural communication in UK maternity services: A Freedom of Information request. *International Journal of Nursing Studies Advances, 6*, 100162. https://doi.org/10.1016/j.ijnsa.2023.100162

Mannava, P., Durrant, K., Fisher, J., Chersich, M., & Luchters, S. (2015). Attitudes and behaviours of maternal health care providers in interactions with clients: A systematic review. *Globalization and Health, 11*(1), 36. https://doi.org/10.1186/s12992-015-0117-9

Marler, H., & Ditton, A. (2021). "I'm smiling back at you": Exploring the impact of mask wearing on communication in healthcare. *International Journal of Language & Communication Disorders, 56*(1), 205–214. https://doi.org/10.1111/1460-6984.12578

Marsh, A., Hundley, V., Luce, A., & Richens, Y. (2023a). What are UK nurses and midwives' views and experiences of using social media within their role? A review. *MIDIRS Midwifery Digest, 33*(4), 312–318.

Marsh, A., Hundley, V., Luce, A., & Richens, Y. (2023b). The perfect birth: a content analysis of midwives' posts about birth on Instagram. *BMC Pregnancy and Childbirth, 23*(1), 422. https://doi.org/10.1186/s12884-023-05706-2

Marsh, A., & Lowry, D. (2023). *The TikTok labour and delivery nurse - A case study*. Retrieved false18/01/2024 from https://www.all4maternity.com/the-tiktok-labour-and-delivery-nurse-a-case-study/

Marsh, A., Ward, S., Collins, S., Milnes, A., Sinaga, K., Smith, H., & Welford, C. (2024). Ask a midwife - A service evaluation. *The Practising Midwife, 27*(2), 40–43.

McCann, E., Brown, M., Hollins-Martin, C., Murray, K., & McCormick, F. (2021). The views and experiences of LGBTQ+ people regarding midwifery care: A systematic review of the international evidence. *Midwifery, 103*, 103102. https://doi.org/10.1016/j.midw.2021.103102

McCarthy, R., Byrne, G., Brettle, A., Choucri, L., Ormandy, P., & Chatwin, J. (2020). Midwife-moderated social media groups as a validated information source for women during pregnancy. *Midwifery, 88*, 102710. https://doi.org/10.1016/j.midw.2020.102710

McCarthy, R., Choucri, L., Ormandy, P., & Brettle, A. (2017). Midwifery continuity: The use of social media. *Midwifery, 52*, 34–41. https://doi.org/10.1016/j.midw.2017.05.012

Menage, D., Bailey, E., Lees, S., & Coad, J. (2020). Women's lived experience of compassionate midwifery: Human and professional. *Midwifery, 85*, 102662. https://doi.org/10.1016/j.midw.2020.102662

Ménage, D., Bailey, E., Lees, S., & Coad, J. (2017). A concept analysis of compassionate midwifery. *Journal of Advanced Nursing, 73*(3), 558–573. https://doi.org/10.1111/jan.13214

Mirzaee, F., & Dehghan, M. (2020). A model of trust within the mother-midwife relationship: A grounded theory approach. *Obstetrics and Gynecology International, 2020,* 9185313. https://doi.org/10.1155/2020/9185313

Morse, H., & Brown, A. (2022a). The benefits, challenges and impacts of accessing social media group support for breastfeeding: A systematic review. *Maternal & Child Nutrition, 18*(4), e13399. https://doi.org/10.1111/mcn.13399

Morse, H., & Brown, A. (2022b). Mothers' experiences of using Facebook groups for local breastfeeding support: Results of an online survey exploring midwife moderation. *PLOS Digit Health, 1*(11), e0000144. https://doi.org/10.1371/journal.pdig.0000144

Morse, H., & Brown, A. (2023). UK midwives' perceptions and experiences of using Facebook to provide perinatal support: Results of an exploratory online survey. *PLOS Digit Health, 2*(4), e0000043. https://doi.org/10.1371/journal.pdig.0000043

National Maternity Review Team. (2016). *Better births – Improving outcomes of maternity services in England.* https://www.england.nhs.uk/wp-content/uploads/2016/02/national-maternity-review-report.pdf

NHS England. (2023). *Three year delivery plan for maternity and neonatal services.* https://www.england.nhs.uk/wp-content/uploads/2023/03/B1915-three-year-delivery-plan-for-maternity-and-neonatal-services-march-2023.pdf

Ockenden, D. (2022). *Final report of the Ockenden review. Findings, conclusions and essential actions from the independent review of maternity services at the Shrewsbury and Telford Hospital NHS Trust.* Department of Health and Social Care. https://www.gov.uk/government/publications/final-report-of-the-ockenden-review

Papadopoulos, I., Lazzarino, R., Koulouglioti, C., Aagard, M., Akman, Ö., Alpers, L. M., Apostolara, P., Araneda Bernal, J., Biglete-Pangilinan, S., Eldar-Regev, O., González-Gil, M. T., Kouta, C., Krepinska, R., Lesińska-Sawicka, M., Liskova, M., Lopez-Diaz, A. L., Malliarou, M., Martín-García, Á., Muñoz-Salinas, M., Nagórska, M., … Zorba, A. (2020). Obstacles to compassion-giving among nursing and midwifery managers: An international study. *International Nursing Review, 67*(4), 453–465. https://doi.org/10.1111/inr.12611

Perez-Botella, M., Downe, S., Magistretti, C. M., Lindstrom, B., & Berg, M. (2015). The use of salutogenesis theory in empirical studies of maternity care for healthy mothers and babies. *Sexual & Reproductive Healthcare: Official Journal of the Swedish Association of Midwives, 6*(1), 33–39. https://doi.org/10.1016/j.srhc.2014.09.001

Royal College of Midwives. (2016). *Why midwives leave – Revisited.* https://cdn.ps.emap.com/wp-content/uploads/sites/3/2016/10/Why-Midwives-Leave.pdf

Royal College of Midwives. (2021). *The solution – Series 2: Making maternity services safer: The role of leadership.* https://www.rcm.org.uk/media/5064/the-solution-series-2-making-maternity-services-safer-the-role-of-leadership.pdf

Royal College of Midwives. (2022). *The re:birth project, final report.* https://www.rcm.org.uk/media/6327/rebirth-final-full-report-july-2022.pdf

Sandall, J., Soltani, H., Gates, S., Shennan, A., & Devane, D. (2016). Midwife-led continuity models versus other models of care for childbearing women. *Cochrane Database of Systematic Reviews, 4.* https://doi.org/10.1002/14651858.CD004667.pub5

Sanders, R. A., & Crozier, K. (2018). How do informal information sources influence women's decision-making for birth? A meta-synthesis of qualitative studies. *BMC Pregnancy and Childbirth, 18*(1), 21. https://doi.org/10.1186/s12884-017-1648-2

Sist, L., Savadori, S., Grandi, A., Martoni, M., Baiocchi, E., Lombardo, C., & Colombo, L. (2022). Self-care for nurses and midwives: Findings from a scoping review. *Healthcare (Basel)*, *10*(12). https://doi.org/10.3390/healthcare10122473

Stapleton, H., Kirkham, M., & Thomas, G. (2002). Qualitative study of evidence based leaflets in maternity care. *BMJ*, *324*(7338), 639. https://doi.org/10.1136/bmj.324.7338.639

Solhaug, I., de Vibe, M., Friborg, O., Sorlie, T., Tyssen, R., Bkorndal, A., & Rosenvinge, J. (2019). Long-term mental health effects of mindfulness training: A 4-year follow-up study. *Mindfulness*, *10*, 1661–1672. https://doi.org/10.1007/s12671-019-01100-2

Vranceanu, A.-M., Elbon, M., Adams, M., & Ring, D. (2012). The emotive impact of medical language. *The Hand*, *7*(3), 293–296. https://doi.org/10.1007/s11552-012-9419-z

Watson, K., White, C., Hall, H., & Hewitt, A. (2021). Women's experiences of birth trauma: A scoping review. *Women and Birth: Journal of the Australian College of Midwives*, *34*(5), 417–424. https://doi.org/10.1016/j.wombi.2020.09.016

Weyant, R. A., Clukey, L., Roberts, M., & Henderson, A. (2017). Show your stuff and watch your tone: Nurses' caring behaviors. *American Journal of Critical Care*, *26*(2), 111–117. https://doi.org/10.4037/ajcc2017462

Young, M. E., Norman, G. R., & Humphreys, K. R. (2008). The role of medical language in changing public perceptions of illness. *PLoS One*, *3*(12), e3875. https://doi.org/10.1371/journal.pone.0003875

7

LOVE AS TIME

Diane Ménage and Jenny Patterson

Society and time

Our modern view of time has only been around for the last 200 years or so. Pre-industrialisation (when most work was home based), the passage of time was noted through the seasons and the natural cycles of day and night, for example, how high the sun was in the sky. Although clocks of sorts had been around for many hundreds of years, most homes would not have had a clock until well into the nineteenth century when there was the means to mass produce them. With industrialisation came the need to organise people and services. Working days needed to bring people together, for example in a factory to keep machines and processes running. The coming of organised transport, particularly the railways, required exacting notions of time to enable reliable timetables. Our current 24/7 society values speed, fast broadband, fast cars, high speed trains, fast food, and so on; we need to work faster or complete more work by continuing through breaks and over hours. Work spills over into home life. We refer to the *rat race*, the *rush hour*. As people, we are pushed to do more in less time, to be efficient. Time is money! Midwifery, as a human, societal occupation, reflects and contributes to values in society. The consideration of time as money is pertinent to midwifery in terms of hospital and maternity unit bed spaces, and fast turnover is needed to ensure more women can be admitted when needed.

Midwifery and time

As maternity services became organised within hospitals in the 1960s, shift patterns and timings became the norm for midwives. Not only to organise the

DOI: 10.4324/9781032645780-10

work force but to monitor birthing women and their babies. We ask women and their partners to *time* contractions and phone triage or attend the maternity unit when they meet a certain frequency or length. We continue to measure the timing of contractions as well as length of different stages of labour, particularly second and third stages. This has become the norm. Thus, as midwives, much of our time is spent *doing* things such as timing, counting, measuring, estimating, documenting, planning, and referring activities, which all increase when complications are present (Browne & Chandra, 2009). In the name of safety, efficiency, and speed, we are continually being pushed to *do* more and more.

It is easy to think that this has always been the case and forget that in the natural world, time is not measured and managed in the same way. To ask when the baby will be born is like asking a farmer when the crop will be ready for harvest. Midwives live with this conceptual contradiction on a day-to-day basis. We know that physiological birth is part of the natural world and cannot be controlled by timings and yet we work in environments that are governed by the clock. We also know that attaching specific *time* expectations or assessments are not appropriate for every woman; individual physiology may not be considered or acknowledged.

A lack of love?

We suggest that this approach is also not *loving*, through a lack of individual focus. However, balancing an appreciation for such natural rhythms with the demands of modern life and maternity care systems is something that midwives must try to do every day. Importantly, the focus on processes that rely on suboptimal technologies takes us away from being able to wait, trust, and support the physiological processes of human birth that evidence tells us can improve outcomes for women and babies (Buckley, 2015). There are times, such as during obstetric complications, where speed is of the essence in midwifery. Yet, the concern here is when fast is valued over slow, where the systems we work within value efficiency over relationships. Furthermore, this pressure to *do*, to achieve, to tick boxes, leaves little time to *be with*, to build the relationships that women and midwives desire and need, let alone valuing and loving these relationships (Browne & Chandra, 2009; Patterson et al., 2019). Midwives have a conflicting relationship with time; they need to be authentically present and *with woman* in-the-moment, but at the same time, they need to anticipate what complications might happen and to do this they need to consider the future. Arguably, this ability to stay in the moment with the woman and yet plan for different possible futures is one of the hallmarks of a good midwife. There is also conflict between midwives' aspiration of truly *being* with women and the institutional expectations of the role which prioritises the *doing* aspect of the job and this is a major factor compromising midwives' emotional wellbeing and leading to job dissatisfaction (Leinweber & Rowe, 2010; Patterson et al., 2019).

The drive to achieve more

This drive to achieve more is reflected by one of the most common complaints from midwives: that there is not enough time to care for women and families in the way that they would like to. While a heavy and ever-increasing workload is key, this is compounded by lack of staff. These issues have certainly been heightened in recent years and particularly during and since the COVID-19 pandemic. Nevertheless, it is worth noting that this is not a new problem. It is difficult to think of any period in the last few decades when this has not been expressed as a concern and it can be argued that not having enough time has been an ongoing feature of most current maternity workers' professional lives. During a 2005 conference entitled *A Labour of Love? Emotion Work and Reproduction*, time was referred to as a source of oppression for midwives due to "temporal pressure, unpredictability, and rapid turnover" (Seekings-Norman, 2005, p. 16). Moreover, women and families have complained that they were not given enough time with midwives. For example, they have reported that they were left alone in labour or that the midwives did not have time to provide breastfeeding support (Lawlor et al., 2023). Even for women who have not named these sorts of issues, one thing that most service-users will remember is that the midwives were very busy. Somehow, *busyness* has become almost synonymous with midwifery work. Many of us have often heard women say, "I didn't like to ask her or bother her [the midwife], she was so busy."

The effect of such busyness

Such busyness can be problematic. Firstly, for the women and families who feel that they cannot bother a midwife who is busy. This has a knock-on effect: they are reluctant to ask the midwife questions or ask for help, they may not disclose that they are feeling unwell, frightened, or depressed, they do not seek support with breastfeeding…the list goes on. The problems do not go away, they are just stacking up, ready to erupt in another way. Problems that should have been picked up and resolved are missed and become more acute, women and their families get upset or angry, and complaints increase. There is a point at which busyness is inefficient and even dangerous. Secondly, being too busy is problematic for midwives. Findings from a United Kingdom survey stated that the "overwhelming impression was that many midwives felt exhausted by their day-to-day work" (Hunter et al., 2017, p. 15) with two thirds thinking about leaving the profession. The main reasons given for considering leaving were poor staffing levels, concerns with the quality of care, and dissatisfaction with organisation of care, with many midwives reporting that they do not get any cover for breaks.

These concerns are not just a problem in the UK; they are features of midwifery in many parts of the world (Carvajal et al., 2024). While midwives in low-income countries experience many difficulties that midwives in high-income countries do not encounter, midwives' working conditions are universally challenging with poor staffing levels and high intensity widely reported. When these conditions are combined with the responsibilities involved in the midwife's role, it is evident that midwives' working conditions can be very difficult. While the severity of the problem on an objective measurable level differs between countries and models of care, the subjective perception of lack of time appears to be universal. Referring to subjective perception is not to suggest lack of time is not real because it absolutely is, rather it illustrates the complexity of this issue of *lack of time*. There is no one solution to this and any possible solution would itself require time to make an impact. Meanwhile, midwives today need to navigate suboptimal working environments now and a good place to start could be exploring the concept of time and how we think of it.

So, let's slow down, perhaps even stop for a moment, and take time to reflect.

Time is finite

The problem with time is that it is finite. We can never get any more; we can only have it one moment at a time. We only have *now* and everything else is the past or the future. We understand time as being a continuous, measurable, precise, and predictable entity. However, it is worth taking a broader view of time. For example, different cultures may have distinct concepts and expressions related to time. Some cultures place a strong emphasis on punctuality, while others may have a more relaxed attitude towards time. Illustrative examples include that of the Kilimanjaro mountain guide who says *polepole* (a Swahili word pronounced *PollyPolly* and meaning slowly, slowly) is the way to climb a mountain (Moshi, 2016). Another example is the story, also referred to in Chapter 9, of an explorer pushing his porters to go faster, to not waste a minute, only to find that they all stopped, explaining "we have been moving very quickly so we have left our souls behind, we need to wait for them to catch up with us again" (Cuevas, 2022).

Time as a language of love in midwifery

To explore time as a love language in midwifery, we can reflect that midwives want to provide high-quality care. As discussed in earlier chapters, we believe that practising from a place of love is the motivation and hallmark of such care. However, lack of time may be experienced as a barrier to practising lovingly. Given that the problem of not enough time is complex and persistent, it is not going to be a quick fix. Within midwifery, two key issues that impact on time are heavy workload and staffing shortages; these are now explored.

While much can be done to improve the very real staffing shortages, and medium-to-long-term planning must aim to do this, maternity care is unpredictable by nature and there will always be periods when a midwife's time is stretched. Midwifery staffing is a complex task in many ways, not least because admissions fluctuate considerably, and the timing of birth cannot be predicted. Therefore, an important and practical approach would be to explore concepts such as midwife/woman ratios and whether midwives are spending their time on the right things. We discovered that there is an astonishing lack of evidence regarding how many midwives are needed. Indeed, the UK's National Institute for Health and Care Excellence (NICE) guidance on safe staffing levels has not been reviewed since 2015 (NICE, 2015). There are tools which can be used to guide safe staffing and one example is Birthrate Plus (Ball et al., n.d.), the tool of choice in the UK. However, it lacks a robust evidence base (Griffiths et al., 2024) and while based on activity and complexity, it does not effectively assist with understanding the time needed to provide care across complex and varied intrapartum scenarios. Furthermore, Griffiths et al. (2024) highlight a lack of published evidence of updates to the tool, a concern given that clearly there have been some changes to midwives' workload and responsibilities since it was developed.

There are also very few studies on how midwives spend their time, and it is surprising that more research and development has not been carried out into this task. One key area of change has been documentation, which has increased over the years. Cooper et al. (2021) demonstrated that midwives spend 21–28% of their time on documentation tasks and that there are numerous frustrations with duplication which contribute to a feeling that documentation is taking too much time and distracts from actual care. Electronic records have been introduced into many areas with the promise of improving this situation, and while there have been advantages it has not improved the workload for all, with some midwives struggling to reconcile being *with woman* and being *with computer* (Hadland et al., 2022). However, faced with the new reality of electronic records, midwives do develop ways to negotiate these competing demands, practising lovingly by prioritising being with woman while also fulfilling their professional requirement to complete records. These words from an experienced UK midwife provide an example of this:

> I am slow on the computer records that we have to do. It is frustrating and I see that the younger generation are much faster than me. But I support the woman and give the care. So, for example, if I am looking after someone in the second stage of labour, I concentrate on giving the care and then document afterwards. I think I would never get top marks for documentation for that very reason. I note the observations and things as they happen...but I complete the computer records after the care. I care for the woman and then after the delivery, nine times out of ten I am doing my documentation

for an hour afterwards! I always say to the woman: I am not ignoring you and just let me know if you need anything, but I just have to do the documentation now. The women want a midwife that supports them first and foremost. We are not going to get it right for everybody and I have to accept that too. But my instinct is to always try to give the best care I can. Eilish, Labour Ward Midwife, UK.

While acknowledging the very real practical considerations of workload and staffing issues that may never be fully resolved, how can we as midwives be creative and loving in the way we use time? How can time become a language of love in midwifery?

Giving time lovingly in midwifery

One way to look at the problem is to be clear about what aspects of the work are most important to us, using love as a value to guide practice. Most midwives come into the profession to provide high-quality, compassionate care to women and families; to make a positive difference. Using love as a value allows us to focus on this vision as a priority, so that whatever we do, we are focussed on doing it lovingly. This is not just great for those we care for; but as discussed in Chapter 1, it feels good to do things with love!

At the heart of midwifery, we have the midwife–mother relationship (Kirkham, 2010). We know that this relationship is central to the childbearing experience and midwifery care, and that both midwives and women desire a positive, compassionate relationship (Menage et al., 2020; Patterson et al., 2019). But over and above aesthetics, a positive relationship where midwives *hold space* and enable birth to *unfold* is key to optimising the physiological and psychological processes of childbirth (Browne & Chandra, 2009; Buckley, 2015). As discussed throughout this book, relationship and connection can be seen as the vehicles for loving midwifery practice. If time is a language of love, then as midwives for whom love is at the heart of our relationships with the women and families we care for, how can we use our time in the best way, within complex systems that have all but forgotten the need to give time?

We now explore some approaches that could help us use our time lovingly in midwifery.

Connection

While continuity of carer models hold potential for spending more time with women, loving practice can be demonstrated in any model of care moment-by-moment. Many midwives are experts at striking up a connection and kick-starting a trusting relationship with the women in their care, even when they have never met them before. What is more, women look out for this and very quickly notice midwives' attentiveness and willingness to connect, sometimes within a few seconds of meeting them, and they highly value this (Menage et al., 2020). Practising lovingly is always about connection – connection with those we care for, our colleagues, and ourselves. The danger is that when midwives feel they are rushed off their feet (not enough time or staff) or do not have enough headspace (too many competing demands), this important way of connecting skilfully and lovingly with women can be diminished or even lost. Worryingly, the current UK NHS maternity care culture that upholds a *keep going* attitude (next woman, next shift...) does not value a culture of *presence*, the being with women that facilitates physiological birth processes (Tabib et al., 2024). Yet, it is possible to reclaim time for connection and relationship. It is not all about having more time, it is also about how we use our time. Time as a love language is about quality over quantity (University of Arizona Global Campus, 2021). Quality time in midwifery is giving undivided attention, practising active listening, in other words being present, using a loving approach. Elizabeth's words below are a good example of quality over quantity when it comes to giving time:

> More time is not always the answer. You can save a lot of time by getting to the crux of what the woman needs quickly. It's about being present. If your head is full of your own stuff or just thinking about what you want to say, you are not being present. It's about giving people your full attention and picking up all the cues...and I want to do that because I am interested in people, and I actually do care. Elizabeth, Midwife UK.

Slow midwifery

So, what might it mean to slow down in midwifery? Perhaps we need to reconnect with our humanness, to reflect on that which we instinctively know, demonstrated by expressions such as *catch my breath*; *take a moment*; *more haste, less speed*; and *one step at a time*. Moving faster and faster is not sustainable as a regular way of life or work. The human need to slow down or *let our souls catch up* is reflected by an ongoing global trend towards valuing *slow* (slow food, slow cities, slow parenting) (Browne & Chandra, 2009; Honoré, n.d.). The purpose of slowing down is to achieve a better quality or balance within life. Taking this approach in midwifery may enable midwives to become and remain connected to women and less connected to our schedules and clocks. Although in current maternity systems it is unlikely there will be more time to provide midwifery care, our sense of time and how we use it is as much in our minds as it is practical. Also, we suggest that being fully present to someone might not require more time but rather a more loving focus.

How midwives might be able to adjust the way they think of and relate to time has been explored by Tabib et al. (2024). They found that midwives commented on bringing a culture of presence into their practice that was perceived to be at odds with the current culture within the maternity service. This culture of practice was regarded as conducive to "facilitating childbirth physiological processes and preventing the midwife from intervening unnecessarily" (Tabib et al., 2024, p. 5). We consider such a culture of presence to be a loving approach which has potential to optimise physiological outcomes. Furthermore, and crucially, if we extend this loving approach and presence towards our colleagues, then the time wasted in tense toxic environments could be reduced, as one midwife participant in Patterson et al. (2019) said "if we just supported each other, and looked out for each other, and worked as a team…half the nonsense would go, and we would actually have more time" (p. 26).

Emotional intelligence

A study by Tabib et al. (2024) found that for midwives to be mentally and emotionally present to a woman's psychological needs, whilst meeting the institutional demands, they require high levels of emotional intelligence (EI). EI has been defined as a set of skills that enable individuals to recognise, understand, and manage their own emotions, as well as the emotions of others (Goleman, 1996). See Box 7.1 for an interesting reflection about EI in midwives. Tabib et al. (2024) introduced EI education to a small group of midwives and the findings show that changing our mindset and awareness through relaxation makes it possible to alter the perception of busyness and the need to keep doing. They found that by *stepping back* from being the *thinker* to become the *observer*, midwives can recognise their own stress and through self-relaxation "just take a breath and calm down," which can take them from feeling stressed to feeling calm (Tabib et al., 2024, p. 3). This move to calmness enabled midwives to become present to women, and to connect and be *with woman* thus alleviating her stress, while protecting their own emotional wellbeing. This formed part of the theme "A different approach to practice" which resulted in a positive "ripple effect" towards women and colleagues. Embracing this approach enabled midwives to "make the most of little pockets of time…with the woman…taking that moment together…explore how she is feeling…not so willing to jump in and tell them what to do," and midwives found they wanted to spend more time and "not be in such a rush" (Tabib et al., 2024, p. 7). One midwife participant identified a real sense of change in mindset:

> So, instead of being like, oh, I just want to get this visit over and done with, I've got all this extra stuff to do, it's been quite nice to be like, actually, I want to take a longer time, I want to sit with this woman, which is so then I'm getting a bit more job satisfaction.
>
> *(Tabib et al., 2024, p. 5)*

BOX 7.1 REFLECTION ON "RECIPE FOR BEING A MIDWIFE" (AUTHOR UNKNOWN)

2 heaped cups full of patience
1 heart full of love
2 handfuls of generosity
1 head full of understanding, and a dash of humour
Sprinkle with kindness and plenty of faith, and mix well
Spread over a lifetime's work as a midwife, and serve to every childbearing woman, partner, baby, and family.

This recipe was told to me as a student midwife. It is a heartfelt and warm narrative that I believe captures the need for a midwife to possess emotional intelligence (EI) to a level that enhances care provision at a holistic level, which includes providing quality psychological and social elements of care adjacent to the physical. EI includes ability to comprehend, utilise, and manage self-emotions alongside the emotions of others. Within the midwife's role, these elements are brought to life in relationships with childbearing women, infants, partners, families, and peer members of the maternity care team. Holding an enhanced EI can help the midwife build stronger relationships, have greater success at work, and achieve goals to a high level. Domains of EI include self-awareness, self-regulation, motivation, empathy, social awareness, and quality relationship management. Together these elements of EI help the midwife face events with reduced stress and emotional reactivity, which incurs fewer unintended consequences. Midwives who possess a high EI can walk in another person's moccasins, and by doing so understand what they are going through. The recipe for a midwife is a simple, humorous, and creative way of capturing these.

Reflection written by Professor Caroline Joy Hollins Martin, 1st November 2024.

Interestingly, this echoes Adib-Hajbaghery and BolandianBafghi (2020) who consider the allocation of sufficient time for patient care to be a result of love in nursing. These moves towards calmness, slowing down, and spending more time with, all help develop the patience, generosity, and understanding described in Box 7.1.

Allocating time in a more loving way

While the work by Tabib et al. (2024) shows it is possible to rethink how we use our time as midwives, there is also a need to change how we prioritise the

---

BOX 7.2   DISTRESS DUE TO SENSE OF ABANDONMENT AFTER BIRTH (PATTERSON ET AL., 2019)

It's very frustrating if you've looked after a woman, delivered her baby and you have no time afterwards with them at all (...) I think that that's the one I find the worst (Midwife, p. 26).

...bounced from one room once the placenta's out, shoved into another room (...) completely abandoned that woman (Midwife, p. 26).

I felt like they were done with me um yeah the baby was born the baby was fine and I didn't really matter (...) right we've done her she's okay, next one (Woman, p. 31).

---

allocation of time. The current approach in most UK maternity care settings prioritises physical wellbeing but does not extend this to psychological wellbeing. When a woman arrives at a maternity unit in labour, she will be allocated as much time as is needed until her baby is born and the placenta delivered. This could be 30 minutes or 48 hours, the point is that the allocation of a midwife will remain, albeit with shift changes, up to this point. However, after the placenta is delivered, often the midwife is reallocated rather than remaining with the woman during the first hour or two after birth. This is a serious problem. Much of the psychological trauma and subsequent post-traumatic stress disorder that exists is due to a sense of abandonment directly after the birth, as expressed by participants from a study exploring distressing aspects of interaction between women and midwives (See box 7.2).

If the allocation of sufficient time is the result of love, then a fully loving approach would encompass psychological wellbeing and ensure that the continuation of the midwife's presence with the woman is supported to extend into the first hours after birth. This would reflect a truly holistic and loving approach within midwifery and optimise both physical and psychological outcomes, thereby reducing the human suffering and systemic costs that arise following psychological trauma.

Sustainability

To use time lovingly within midwifery, midwives need to sustain their own wellbeing. While midwives can, and perhaps should, be involved in taking action to push for safe staffing levels and seeking solutions to workload demands, maternity services have a responsibility to take care of midwives. This is explored more fully in Chapters 9 and 10. Nevertheless, to practise more lovingly within complex and pressured systems midwives need to be able to cope with the situations they find themselves in now, today. Here, we introduce a few suggestions and considerations that may be beneficial in managing the alarming feelings around being very busy and there not being enough time. Chapter 9 provides more discussion on this topic.

Mindfulness techniques such as those developed by Gilbert (2009) and Puddicombe (2016) can provide a way of feeling connected in the here and now. Not with our thoughts and actions but with the essence of ourselves and our common humanity. While there are many techniques to assist with this, most utilise the body to bring our attention to the present moment. Focusing on our breath is one of the most common methods. Noticing the *in* and the *out* breath with curiosity can help bring a moment of calm. Thoughts will come into our mind because that is what our minds do, it is to be expected. Mindfulness techniques help us to practise acknowledging these thoughts, while not being led by them; instead coming back to focus on our breath. The great thing about mindfulness is that even if only used for a few minutes or seconds, it can be helpful. Mindfulness is a practice, and it needs to be *practised* but it is not a case of getting *good at it* or *doing it right*.

In an imperfect environment, things will sometimes (through no one's fault) be imperfect. Developing skills around prioritisation, appropriate delegation and effective time management are essential but they can only go so far. When there is not enough time to care in the way they would wish to, midwives start to feel dissatisfied with their work and become self-critical of the things they did not do well or that they forgot. While reflection on practice and supportive, constructive criticism can be positive aids to learning, this is not the same as harsh or destructive self-criticism. This sort of self-criticism serves no useful purpose because it focuses on blame and guilt rather than learning and moving forward. Rather than (unhelpful) self-criticism, we need self-compassion. Mindfulness and self-compassion are closely linked. Kristin Neff (2024) has developed a body of work on this topic including mindful self-compassion techniques. Neff explains that self-compassion has three elements: self-kindness, connectedness, and mindfulness. All three elements are applicable in midwifery and a model showing actions and intentions for midwives and other maternity care workers, based on these elements, has recently been developed (Byrom et al., n.d.). Self-compassion is one form of self-love and Chapter 9 discusses other aspects and discusses love for self in depth.

Another crucial skill required to maintain loving practice is that of *setting boundaries*. While midwifery professional bodies provide guidance on professional boundaries, setting our own boundaries as employees and human beings is necessary to sustain loving care of ourselves and others (see Chapter 13 for further discussion on boundaries). As discussed earlier, it has become a normal, often accepted part of the culture, to miss breaks. This will contravene working time directives in many countries, e.g., in the UK anybody who works longer than six hours is entitled to an uninterrupted break by law. Yet, many UK midwives work long shifts of ten hours or more and are not paid for their meal break (whether they take it or not) and often they do not. It is essential that we move away from this damaging culture and ensure that we do have our breaks.

As midwives, we can be very good at advocating for those we care for, but we need to get a whole lot better at advocating for ourselves. Self-love, explored more fully in Chapter 9, should be at the heart of this and good communication skills and assertiveness will assist. Midwives can bring these practices and skills into play in order to learn how to say no when unfair burdens are placed upon them, and when they need to escalate concerns about excessive workloads and to protect their own wellbeing (Hazard, 2021); it is encouraging that these skills are increasingly being introduced in under-graduate nursing and midwifery programmes (Hanson et al., 2020; Lee et al., 2023; Warland et al., 2014).

Conclusion

As midwives, we sometimes experience tremendous pressure to achieve a lot in a very short space of time. Workplace conditions such as staffing levels, access to breaks, as well as workplace culture have a significant impact on how we are able to use time lovingly with those we provide care for and our colleagues. We have explored concepts such as connection, slow midwifery, emotional intelli-gence, boundary setting, mindfulness, and self-compassion as approaches that might help us use time as a language of love in midwifery. We have briefly out-lined some suggestions for self-care that will enable us to sustain this loving practice.

References

Adib-Hajbaghery, M., & BolandianBafghi, S. (2020). Love in nursing: A concept anal-ysis. *Journal of Caring Sciences, 9*(2), 113–119. https://doi.org/10.34172/JCS.2020.017

Ball, J. A., Washbrook, M., & The Royal College of Midwives. (n.d.). *Birthrate plus R: What it is and why you should be using it.* https://www.rcm.org.uk/media/2367/birthrate-plus-what-it-is-and-why-you-should-be-using-it.pdf

Browne, J., & Chandra, A. (2009). Slow midwifery. *Women and Birth: Journal of the Australian College of Midwives, 22*(1), 29–33. https://doi.org/10.1016/j.wombi.2008.10.003

Buckley S. J. (2015). Executive summary of hormonal physiology of childbearing: Evidence and implications for women, babies, and maternity care. *The Journal of Perinatal Education, 24*(3), 145–153. https://doi.org/10.1891/1058-1243.24.3.145

Byrom, S., Ménage, D., & Patterson, J. (n.d.). Compassion as a cure – Humanising midwifery work. In E. Newnham, L. McKellar, Mayra, K., & Kuipers, K. (Eds.), *Humanising birth – Solutions for the global maternity crisis.* Springer Nature.

Carvajal, B., Hancock, A., Lewney, K., Hagan, K., Jamieson, S., & Cooke, A. (2024). A global overview of midwives' working conditions: A rapid review of literature on positive practice environment. *Women and Birth: Journal of the Australian College of Midwives, 37(*1), 15–50. https://doi.org/10.1016/j.wombi.2023.08.007

Cooper, A. L., Brown, J. A., Eccles, S. P., Cooper, N., & Albrecht, M. A. (2021). Is nursing and midwifery clinical documentation a burden? An empirical study of perception versus reality. *Journal of Clinical Nursing, 30*(11–12), 1645–1652. https://doi.org/10.1111/jocn.15718

Cuevas, G.S. (2022). *Take a moment for your soul to catch up with you: A beautiful African story.* https://exploringyourmind.com/moment-your-soul-to-catch-up-beautiful-african-story/

Gilbert, P. (2009) *The compassionate mind.* Constable and Robinson.

Goleman, D. (1996). *Emotional intelligence: 25th anniversary edition.* Bloomsbury Publishing Plc.

Griffiths, P., Turner, L., Lown, J., & Sanders, J. (2024). Evidence on the use of birthrate plus® to guide safe staffing in maternity services – A systematic scoping review. *Women and Birth: Journal of the Australian College of Midwives, 37*(2), 317–324. https://doi.org/10.1016/j.wombi.2023.11.003

Hadland, M., Smyth, W., Craswell, A., Kearney, L., & Nagle, C. (2022). O50 - Being with computer: Midwives' perspectives of the impact of the electronic maternity record on their practice providing woman-centred care. *Women & Birth, 35*(Suppl 1), 20. https://doi.org/10.1016/j.wombi.2022.07.056

Hanson, J., Walsh, S., Mason, M., Wadsworth, D., Framp, A., & Watson, K. (2020). 'Speaking up for safety': A graded assertiveness intervention for first year nursing students in preparation for clinical placement: Thematic analysis. *Nurse Education Today, 84*, 104252. https://doi.org/10.1016/j.nedt.2019.104252

Hazard, L. (2021). *Surviving in today's NHS: What student midwives need to know. Maternity and Midwifery Forum.* https://maternityandmidwifery.co.uk/surviving-in-todays-nhs/

Honoré, C. (n.d.). *Education and parenting.* https://www.carlhonore.com/education-parenting/

Hunter, B., Henley, J., Fenwick, J., & Sidebotham, M. (2017). *Work, health and emotional lives of midwives in the United Kingdom: The UK WHELM study.* https://www.rcm.org.uk/media/2924/work-health-and-emotional-lives-of-midwives-in-the-united-kingdom-the-uk-whelm-study.pdf

Kirkham, M. (2010). *The midwife-mother relationship* (2nd ed.). Palgrave Macmillan.

Lawlor, N., Prihodova, L., Byrne, D., Etherton, M., Rahill, F., Wilson, C., & O'Sullivan, E. J. (2023). A qualitative analysis of women's postnatal experiences of breastfeeding supports during the perinatal period in Ireland. *PloS One, 18*(7), e0288230. https://doi.org/10.1371/journal.pone.0288230

Lee, S. E., Kim, E., Lee, J. Y., & Morse, B. L. (2023). Assertiveness educational interventions for nursing students and nurses: A systematic review. *Nurse Education Today, 120*, 105655. https://doi.org/10.1016/j.nedt.2022.105655

Leinweber, J., & Rowe, H. J. (2010). The costs of 'being with the woman': secondary traumatic stress in midwifery. *Midwifery, 26*(1), 76–87. https://doi.org/10.1016/j.midw.2008.04.003

Menage, D., Bailey, E., Lees, S., & Coad, J. (2020). Women's lived experience of compassionate midwifery: Human and professional. *Midwifery, 85*, 102662. https://doi.org/10.1016/j.midw.2020.102662

Moshi, W. (2016). Personal communication between J Patterson and Kilimanjaro senior guide and Everest climber. *Wilfred Moshi.*

Neff, K. (2024). *Self compassion.* Dr Kristin Neff Website. https://self-compassion.org/books-by-kristin-neff/

National Institute for Health and Care Excellence (NICE). (2015). *Guideline [NG4] safe midwifery staffing for maternity settings*. https://www.nice.org.uk/guidance/ng4

Patterson, J., Hollins Martin, C. J., & Karatzias, T. (2019). Disempowered midwives and traumatised women: Exploring the parallel processes of care provider interaction that contribute to women developing Post Traumatic Stress Disorder (PTSD) post childbirth. *Midwifery, 76*, 21–35. https://doi.org/10.1016/j.midw.2019.05.010

Puddicombe, A. (2016). *The headspace guide to meditation and mindfulness*. Hodder and Stoughton.

Seekings-Norman, L. (2005). A labour of love? *AIMS Journal, 17*(3), 16. https://www.aims.org.uk/journal/item/a-labour-of-love

Tabib, M., Humphrey, T., & Forbes-McKay, K. (2024). 'Doing' is never enough, if 'being' is neglected. Exploring midwives' perspectives on the influence of an emotional intelligence education programme, a qualitative study. *Women and Birth: Journal of the Australian College of Midwives, 37*(3), 101587. https://doi.org/10.1016/j.wombi.2024.02.003

University of Arizona Global Campus. (2021). *The psychology behind the 5 love languages*. https://www.uagc.edu/blog/the-psychology-behind-the-5-love-languages

Warland, J., McKellar, L., & Diaz, M. (2014). Assertiveness training for undergraduate midwifery students. *Nurse Education in Practice, 14*(6), 752–756. https://doi.org/10.1016/j.nepr.2014.09.006

8

LOVE AS GIFT

Jenny Patterson

Introduction

The *How* is our gift.

The heart of midwifery care rests within the midwife–mother relationship (Kirkham, 2010). There exists a symbiosis between the nature of this relationship and the interaction between each person. Importantly, the perception of the interaction can range from one of compassion (Menage et al., 2020) to one of trauma (Patterson et al., 2019a), emphasising that *how* care is offered is as important as *what* is done. Here, I explore the connection between love, care, and gift in the context of midwifery; the concepts of *Care as Gift* and *Vigil of Care*; and delve into the nature of such *Gift* in terms of what women and midwives desire alongside issues of attitude, power, and sustainability.

Love

Love is the heart of human life. Yet love is as rich and complex as people are diverse and while love can manifest as a powerful, joyful experience, it is often distorted and manipulated, and people suffer. As a cradle Roman Catholic, I have been steeped in teachings about suffering and God's love. Within most faiths, God's love is the energy that flows and unites and keeps the world in being; with an understanding that there exists "a profound unity of love underlying the suffering and brokenness of the world" (Odorisio, 2019, p. 1). I respect that some people will share this understanding, and some will not. Yet, I expect we can agree that as midwives we witness and experience suffering and love every day. While overlap exists with other caring professional relationships, the midwife–mother relationship is unique (Barker, 2011), encompassing love as a

DOI: 10.4324/9781032645780-11

virtue that is "represented by experiencing humanity, human capacity and by a flourishing relationship between human beings – which are at the heart of women centred care...and even keeps midwives in the job at difficult times" (Kuipers, 2022, p. 7). Also, Einion (2023) sees "Midwifery, yes, as love" (p. 7). Furthermore, Oakley (1989) concluded that "love is a scientific concept and its effect on perinatal health can be quantified" (p. 219).

Care and love

Care is defined as "the process of protecting someone...and providing what that person needs" (Cambridge dictionary, 2024) or "responsibility for or attention to health, wellbeing, and safety" (Merriam-Webster, 2024a). If love is a fundamental human emotion, then emotional care must encompass some form of love (Barker, 2011). Eva Luckes, a contemporary of Florence Nightingale and matron of the Royal London Hospital, upheld the rightness of referring to love within care (Mahon, 2016). Love is considered the basis or catalyst for caring, where care is a combination of love and respect and, beautifully, in relation to midwifery, "being with someone towards a moment of joy" (Adib-Hajbaghery & Bolandian Bafghi, 2020, p. 115; Mahon, 2016). Furthermore, Einion (2021) believes midwives are skilled, loving beings "a source of infinite love...who offer love, nurture, support, and excellent clinical safety within a few minutes" (p. 37). Midwives' love and connection with women and families is vital and integral to care (Baston, 2021). Love encompasses respect, dignity, kindness, loyalty, and self-esteem, and includes feelings of attachment, intimacy, and passion, alongside human values, and a sense of goodwill (Adib-Hajbaghery & Bolandian Bafghi, 2020). These are some of the many facets of love, like that of the diamond described in Chapter 2. Importantly, love combines such feelings and values with action through actively seeking reciprocal wellbeing and equality, without conditions (Godden, 2017). Thus, a gift.

Love as gift

Gift is something voluntarily transferred by one person to another without compensation (Merriam Webster, 2024b). The love language of *gift giving* usually refers to tangible items. In midwifery, *gift giving* relates to the benefit that women, families, babies, and colleagues gain from a midwife. Unlike a gift exchange, the gift a midwife offers carries no expectation for return beyond the satisfaction of making a difference (Bolton, 2000). Love often requires choice, choice to be present to the individual, to remain, even in the face of suffering. This choice is our gift to the other. For me, the greatest gift of love was God's gift of His son. Yet not only did God suffer for us, but He suffered *with* us (Odorisio, 2019). This sense of *suffering with* resonates with me as a midwife, in my being *with woman*. When I struggled with the responsibility as an independent midwife, my husband said, "you don't just care for women when they arrive at the station, you board the train and journey with them." Many midwives regardless of their mode of work will relate to this. Many midwives deeply connect with women and families, often to the detriment of their own wellbeing. This choice to *suffer with* and *suffer for* is the heart of the *gift of care* we provide.

Gift, inherent in the expression *giving good care*, requires knowledge and skill alongside close attention to individual need through listening, watching, and touching (Reiger & Lane, 2012). Such actions associated with love languages have been explored in earlier chapters and are evident in the words of women participants from a study exploring experiences of compassionate midwifery care (Menage et al., 2018). Describing the community midwife listening to her when she was struggling with breastfeeding:

> She [the community midwife] was listening more, she was listening first to what I had to say and she was kind of being observant to the situation…and it was like paradise, it was like finally someone that I can, you know, talk to and they can just listen without feeling, I don't know, that they have all the answers…
>
> *Katrin*

Talking about her experience of tenderness from a midwife:

> I think there is something about the tenderness of a touch or the lingering of an eye contact or a squeeze of a hand…the tone of someone's voice that just indicates that they really do get it.
>
> *Mary*

I propose that *Gift* as a love language sits at the very heart of midwifery care.

Vigil of care or care as gift

The terms *Vigil of Care* and *Care as Gift* were first described by Nick Fox in his seminal work on trauma (Fox, 1993, 1995). These terms have been explored within theories around midwifery care and therefore are relevant to explore here.

Firstly, it is important to acknowledge that there has been, and continues to be, much discussion, debate, and even controversy related to differences in care provision approaches between midwifery and medical staff. Both disciplines share a goal of safe and effective care with healthy outcomes. Yet historically, how each has defined care has differed, to the extent of being opposite at times within an often-uneasy collaboration, creating deep-rooted tensions (Oakley, 1989).

This legacy of difference continues to influence the experience, perception, and expectation of care providers today. While we can recognise this, it is not the whole picture. We need a loving approach to look forward and move on in a collaborative, realistic, and sustainable way. Crucially, the following exploration of concepts of care relates to the distinction between the concepts, not between midwives and obstetricians. This is not about *us* and *them*, a concept noted in Chapter 1 and discussed further in Chapters 10 and 13.

Care can be understood as a political process, in which all practitioners try to balance power and expertise, alongside a responsibility to be *caring* over and above action (Fox, 1995). Care can be explored using the concepts of *Vigil of Care* (relating to surveillance using professional expertise and skill) and *Care as Gift* (characterised by trust and generosity, underpinned by love) (Fox, 1995; MacBride-Stewart, 2014; Walsh, 2011). As a means of relating these two concepts to quality of care, it is useful to consider the measurement scale: *Quality of Provider Interaction Inventory* (QPI) (Sorenson, 2003). QPI is a 5-point rating scale that assesses women's perceived quality of interaction with perinatal care providers, their perception of the care provider's verbal and non-verbal behaviour. The QPI scale runs from *disaffirmation* "viewing the person like an object to be assessed, disregarding humanity" (*Vigil of Care* at its worst); to *affirmation* "acknowledging individualised humanity, engaging with and responding to the other" (*Care as Gift* at its best), see Figure 8.1. Disaffirmation is associated with harmful outcomes, while affirmation can facilitate healing (Bedell et al., 2004, Kirkpatrick et al., 2005, as cited in Sorenson & Tschetter, 2010).

Vigilant observation is vital for physical safety, yet *Vigil of Care* can be strongly focussed on risk, surveillance, and intervention, a *technical touch* (El-Nemer et al., 2006). It emphasises care as an institutionalised set of practices through which professionals have the authority to care and to determine

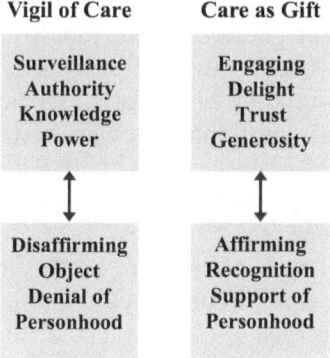

FIGURE 8.1   The parallels that occur between the theories of *Vigil of Care* and *Care as Gift* and the QPI scale.

what it means to care (Bolton et al., 2011). Worryingly, a *Vigil of Care* approach is associated with trauma and distress and is related to poor QPI, with women treated like vessels to be monitored while disregarding human need (Patterson et al., 2019b; Reed et al., 2017). At its worst, *Vigil of Care* links to what is referred to as obstetric violence (El-Nemer et al., 2006), where actions, performed in the name of safety, are ultimately abusive. Patterson et al. (2019b) uncovered scenarios involving coercion through exaggerating risk; physical abuse, including continuation of vaginal examination when the woman, a survivor of rape, repeatedly said stop; and an Entonox mask forcibly held on a woman's face to keep her quiet. El-Nemer et al. (2006) presents violent scenarios including when a woman declined an intervention "the doctor refused and insisted, saying that he is the doctor and he knows what she needs and when, and she must listen to him" (p. 84).

Care as Gift is an approach of openness and mutual respect, it encompasses "generosity, trust, confidence, love, benevolence, commitment, involvement, delight, allegiance, esteem, accord, admiration and curiosity" (Fox, 1993, p. 92). *Care as Gift* is also referred to as "helping from the heart" (El-Nemer et al., 2006, p. 82), favouring the emotional safety of trusting, respectful, loving relationships that align with high-quality QPI where individual personhood is acknowledged (Sorenson, 2003). This location in relationship is central to midwifery care. *Care as Gift* may be exercised as love, trust, and generosity (MacBride-Stewart, 2014), with an awareness of reciprocal belonging and interdependence (Pulcini, 2016), empowering the person who is cared for (Fox, 1995). A recent synthesis and reflection on women-centred care identified 18 virtues, including love, generosity, and compassion (Kuipers, 2022), that resonate with *Care as Gift*. A loving approach to care, far from being a soft option, is fundamental to mothers' satisfaction and babies' health (Oakley, 1989). Midwives' emotion work in navigating the constraints of organisational rules, obligations, and social norms, to be present and to advocate, is clearly a gift (Bolton, 2000; MacBride-Stewart, 2014). Walsh (2011) showcased this beautifully with examples from his ethnographic research of a UK free-standing birth centre. Participants' experiences (Box 8.1) evidence midwives' emotional intelligence (described in Chapter 7) through providing gifts of *presence, time*, and *tuning into need* that, while outside usual care parameters, reveal vital love and human connection and transform individual experience.

Many of us may feel such options are limited in our workplace. Indeed, features of *Care as Gift* may be considered unprofessional and less visible or available to scrutiny than *Vigil of Care* (MacBride-Stewart, 2014). Yet, *Vigil of Care* can undermine the generosity that is inherent within *Care as Gift* (Bolton et al., 2011). Notably, *Vigil of Care* can feel patronising and when someone blindly trusts the *authority* in this care, it can develop more towards dependency (Fox, 1993).

BOX 8.1 PARTICIPANT EXPERIENCES DRAWN FROM WALSH (2011)

One midwife realising that a woman in early labour might benefit from human comfort rather than defaulting to analgesia, chose to spend two hours holding this woman in her arms, on the floor. An open-ended interaction during which the midwife took her lead from the woman.

Another midwife perceived a colleague's needs who had arrived exhausted on shift. She invited and enabled her colleague to have some sleep. Her colleague felt supported and cared for and was able to function better after.

One woman described how, rather than pushing to conform to "normal" timings and patterns, the midwife facilitated her to find her own rhythm, supporting physiological processes and enhancing experience and outcome.

For another woman, anxiety and stress regarding domestic responsibilities were hindering physiological labour. The midwife supported her to go and finish essential Christmas shopping. Acknowledging the woman's need helped her clear the way to progress well in labour on her return.

Today, we consider the midwife–mother relationship to be one of partnership (Hunter, 2006; NMC, 2018). Yet, tensions remain between the responsibility to care for (*Vigil*), while offering *Care as Gift* through being *with woman* and building relationship (MacBride-Stewart, 2014). *Care as gift* is strongly desired by both midwives and women with distress arising when only a humanly disconnected and fragmented *Vigil of Care* is available (Menage et al., 2020; Patterson et al., 2019b).

Care as gift and vigil of care

Perhaps we don't need to choose between *Vigil* or *Gift*, perhaps we can have both, have our cake (many of us love cake!) and eat it. Indeed, this would be the greatest and most loving gift.

Notably, Oakley (1989) said "Love – caring – is as important as science – technical knowledge, monitoring and intervention" (p. 219). Thus, if we (all maternity care professionals) share the same goal, we need care as *Vigil* **and** *Gift*. Skilled, intuitive maternity professionals use their extensive knowledge base while caring for women in a loving way where observation may include watching patiently with love, sensitivity, kindness, attentiveness, understanding, and concern (Bryar & Sinclair, 2011a) referred to as "skilled help from the heart" (El-Nemer et al., 2006, p. 81). Mount (2022) describes midwives as professional friends who dig beyond the medical or alert stickers to share strength, love, support, and a sense of safety, moving beyond *tick boxes* towards wellbeing, joy, elation, and transformation (Bryar & Sinclair, 2011b). Thirty-six years ago, Oakley (1989) called for midwives to do everything to reclaim such a concept of care. More recently, we see that embracing the best of both approaches can improve and maintain safety, while within the context of the midwife–mother relationship, optimising women's experiences of birth (Hunter, 2006; Kirkham, 2010; Patterson et al., 2019b; Reed et al., 2017). By approaching care as both *Vigil* **and** *Gift*, we safeguard both physical and psychological wellbeing for mothers and babies, and subsequently families and wider communities (Ménage & Patterson, 2020), a gift that moves beyond the individual and becomes a commitment towards future generations (Pulcini, 2016).

The nature of gift: the recipient

True gift takes account of the recipient's desires or needs. Women's preferred ways of *doing birth* encompasses warmth, kindness, patience, and feeling emotionally secure, loved, and cherished (El-Nemer et al., 2006). Similarly, across 37 worldwide studies women express a strong desire for "safe, supportive, kind, respectful and responsive care" (Downe et al., 2018, p. 12). Most recently, women describe a positive birth as one when they feel safe, supported, respected, and in control; where they experience joy, confidence, and/or accomplishment, and from which they have a positive impact on their psychosocial wellbeing (Leinweber et al., 2023).

Birth Trauma can result when the reality is far from the desired "safe midwifery embrace" (Baston, 2021, p. 22), not meeting the anticipated "any minute I will be enveloped in a warm welcoming…lovely people will take care of me" (Patterson et al., 2019b, p. 28). Women need midwives who are interested in them, so they can call on them without feeling like a bother, which is central to traumatic birth experiences (Patterson et al., 2019b; Reed et al., 2017). Let's consider Maslow's pyramid (McLeod, 2024), a psychology model comprising five tiers of human needs where needs in the lower tiers must be met before those higher up can be fulfilled. The most fundamental needs are food, water, and safety. Next comes love and belonging. Feeling disregarded or like a nuisance during childbirth, contributes to feeling isolated and unsafe (core aspects of trauma) and fails to meet the need for love and belonging (Adib-Hajbaghery & Bolandian Bafghi, 2020; Baston, 2021), and neglectful or abusive relationships create isolation, distrust, and pain (Lynch, 2007; Patterson et al., 2019b). Women desire the friendly active presence of midwives; to be respected as individuals; to be supported physically and psychologically; to feel safe, secure; and to be able to trust midwives to provide help when they need it, not when midwives think they need it (Barker 2011; Hunter, 2006; Patterson et al., 2019b). Einion (2023) believes midwives bring light in the darkness, offering the gift of removing a sense of burden (feeling like a bother) from women or each other, which is valuable in reducing birth trauma (Patterson et al., 2019b).

The nature of gift: the giver

What motivates us to become midwives? Love is the motivation for care work (Pulcini, 2016) and social work (Perkins, 2022). The compassionate desire to alleviate another person's suffering is a manifestation of human love (Adib-Hajbaghery & Bolandian Bafghi, 2020). Motives include having a sense of vocation or belonging and contributing to a greater good (Moran et al., 2023), while benevolence, generosity, and compassion may arise from sympathy, or empathy (Pulcini, 2016). Midwives' motivations may be complex – on one hand, a motivation to provide loving care to women, babies, and families and make a difference to their experience, on the other, wanting to have a meaningful career, professional status, and earn a living. We want to be viewed as good, caring individuals, to be valued and needed, to be appreciated and validated by women (Hunter, 2006; MacBride-Stewart, 2014). Positive feedback creates joy and job satisfaction; for many midwives, the reward is knowing they have made a difference. Within challenging maternity workplace environments where *Care as Gift* is devalued, such self-interest may enable midwives to find meaning and dignity (Greenstock, 2023; MacBride-Stewart, 2014). Being paid does not prevent us from practising lovingly and creating loving bonds (Pulcini, 2016). In other words, wanting/needing to earn a living does not lessen the fact that we primarily want to make a positive difference to women's experiences. We can create trusting relationships with women and families and practice lovingly, and still with integrity expect to be paid appropriately.

The nature of gift: attitude and power

So, what is the nature of *Care as Gift* rooted in love? How can we provide this within the context of complex maternity care systems? Let's explore attitude and power.

Talking about love in a professional caring context is a marginal not mainstream construct (Godden, 2017). Embracing an attitude of *positive regard* may be more acceptable but what does it mean? When we regard someone, we do more than look, we take account of them in some way. It requires choice to regard positively. Coghlan (2023) refers to taking a *loving look* and that this can enable us to go beyond just knowing, to seeing the value of each individual (as explored in Chapter 1). *Intentional, reflective love* exists within authentic relationship and enables nurse and patient to be truly present to each other (Adib-Hajbaghery & Bolandian Bafghi, 2020). Midwives and nurses contemplate those they provide care for (Coghlan, 2023), where contemplation is defined as taking a long, loving look at the real (Bartunek, 2019). A *loving look* can relate to *benevolent gaze*. The concept of a *benevolent gaze* comes from the writing of Julian of Norwich, a 14th century anchoress and mystic. Julian is well known for her statement "All shall be well, all shall be well, and all manner of things shall be well" drawn from her reflection on the *benevolent gaze* of the divine (Sauro, 2015). Maintaining a benevolent gaze towards women or colleagues, is an attitude of love that fosters positive regard, while *unconditional* positive regard can be understood as a way of truly being with each individual and holding the space for their specific birth experience (Einion, 2021). The word *unconditional* acknowledges that the *real* being contemplated is not always beautiful; midwives are familiar with the ugly, tragic, and sometimes violent aspects of life (Coghlan, 2023). Creating a flourishing relationship in the face of human reality is at the heart of women-centred care through the virtue of love (Kuipers, 2022). Jane describes:

> As a student midwife I cared for a woman in labour who was a substance user; accompanied by her aunt. We provided non-judgemental, compassionate care and managed to create rapport and connection with the woman, despite her deeply rooted fear and distrust of authorities. The woman was enabled to birth well, although her baby was admitted to the neonatal unit with substance withdrawal symptoms. Later the aunt thanked us saying "you were the first people to be kind to my niece in her whole pregnancy.". While pleased, I felt great sadness that perhaps due to anxiety or fear, women in such situations can be judged and not treated with care and respect. Taking a loving approach, gifting the care and attention that we would hope to with everyone, made an important difference.
>
> *Jane: Midwife, UK*

When we choose a loving approach, and *gift* care with compassion, the experience can be positive, even when outcomes are not (Menage et al., 2020). However, when we choose to disregard the human person and forget to look lovingly, then the experience can be traumatic even if clinical outcomes are good (Patterson et al., 2019b). This is a heavy responsibility. Such choice is at the heart of the *Care as Gift* founded on love that I believe is core to midwifery care.

Power exists within relationships (Godden, 2017). The midwife–mother relationship may empower or disempower either party (MacBride-Stewart, 2014). The formal role of midwife carries inherent power, added to by expertise and the weight of policy and guidance. While childbearing can leave women vulnerable and reliant on the care of midwives, women can and do exercise power through choice and consent; whether they show appreciation or not; or using moral and cultural imperatives to demand their care expectations (Lynch, 2007). Embracing the midwife–mother interaction in terms of *other*, or as *us* and *them*, creates a sense of conflict where each person may feel the need to exert their power. To truly listen to and respect the other and then *gift* that which they desire, requires the giver to let go of their own desires or ego. Yet, as midwives, the love we carry in our role can empower us and strengthen our sense of autonomy (Adib-Hajbaghery & Bolandian Bafghi, 2020).

Choosing to adopt a giving attitude, a disposition towards generosity that recognises our own vulnerability and indebtedness to one another, moves away from *us* and *them* (Pulcini, 2016). Compassion can break down barriers and enable us to see what binds us as humans (Peel, 2016). Choosing a loving attitude (love requires choice) enables us to share power, in partnership rather than hierarchy, through openness, listening, and acknowledging the individual (Godden, 2017). Care provided from those with greater power can reduce the recipient's autonomy and include expectations or obligations but can also provide generosity and connection and ultimately be empowering (MacBride-Stewart, 2014).

Love is present within a women-centred approach when midwives take action that empowers women, putting their needs before that of the midwifery profession or the maternity care organisation (Kuipers, 2022; Peel, 2016). This is enabled more easily through continuity of carer (Crowther et al., 2016). Such *gift* is manifest through *stepping back* within the midwife–mother relationship, so the woman is enabled to use her knowledge and make her choices; by respecting and acknowledging the woman we empower her to participate in her care (Kuipers, 2022). This is consistent with the UK Nursing and Midwifery Council (NMC) standard to work in partnership with women (NMC, 2018, Prioritise people, 2.1 & 3.3). This is not a new concept. Oakley (1989) identified midwifery *gift* of care as enabling women and increasing their self-confidence and ability to take control; so, a mother might say "look, we have performed a miracle together: and there was nothing to it!" (p. 220), while 2500 years ago from the Tao Te Ching:

> You are a midwife; you are assisting at someone else's birth.
> Do good without show or fuss.
> Facilitate what is happening rather than what you think ought to be happening.
> If you must take the lead, lead so that the mother is helped yet still free and in charge.
> When the baby is born, the mother will rightly say:
> We did it ourselves!

The nature of gift: sustainability and reciprocity

A study about love in social care describes how community workers are naturally hardwired to give, finding this easier than to receive (Godden, 2017). Undoubtedly, a similar inquiry into midwifery care would conclude this too; we all know midwives who are hardwired to *give* unceasingly. Sometimes the passion and desire to care, the love and generosity within this, motivates midwives to keep giving far beyond their personal resources (Transforming maternity care collaborative, 2024). To sustain such *Care as Gift*, the giver must maintain their personal balance and resources. Many midwives achieve this through their passion for midwifery and joy from supporting childbirth and making a difference to women and families (Crowther et al., 2016). Building meaningful relationships with women keeps work sustainable and satisfying (Hunter, 2006) and is protective (Moran et al., 2023).

And yet, the very nature of immersing ourselves in a midwife–mother relationship demands much of the *giver*. *Care as Gift* is not free, when we *give*, we let go of something, we offer something of ourselves, there is an emotional cost. It is a lifelong struggle to advocate for women, especially those who are marginalised and disempowered (Einion 2021). This emotional cost accumulates and can drain our energy and harm our wellbeing, especially with repeated exposure to trauma (Leinweber & Rowe, 2010), resulting in compassion fatigue "it adds another scar to my soul" (Elmir et al., 2017, p. 4191).

Nevertheless, even with this cost, the love midwives carry for women and midwifery is demonstrated through many stories within this book and beautifully reflected by Godden (2017) where a participant "expressed love through wiping a tear from her eye and rubbing it on the next person's heart" (p. 86). However, such love and giving can mean midwives sacrifice their own wellbeing for the needs of women and suppress their own feelings to maintain an outward appearance that enables women to feel safe (Fitzgerald, 2005 as cited in Adib-Hajbaghery & Bolandian Bafghi, 2020). Such self-sacrifice is a risk factor for poor wellbeing or resilience in midwives (Moran et al., 2023). Loss of wellbeing or low resilience may compromise our ability to be the midwives we desire to be. Thus, applying *Care as Gift* to ourselves (see Chapter 9), contrary to being selfish, is the foundation of sustainable *Care as Gift*. Sustaining healthy resilient midwifery practice where we can lovingly gift care requires self-awareness and self-respect, choosing to pour from a full cup (Greenstock, 2023; Pulcini, 2016). This also enables us to support our colleagues (Lynch, 2007).

Reciprocity refers to exchange or giving between people (Collins English Dictionary, 2024). Billie Hunter (2006) described different types of exchange between women and midwives and the emotional work involved. The nature of gift within midwifery care is not always a balanced exchange. Yes, when rapport, collaboration, and partnership exist, the gift exchange can feel balanced and reciprocal. Yet, the diversity and complexity of human experience may mean our gift is rejected because it is not what the person needs or is able to receive at this time. For example, some women who have experienced interpersonal trauma may find any sort of interaction or relationship difficult (Grossman et al., 2021). When, as midwives, our *Care as Gift* is rejected it can be challenging and increase our emotion work, especially if we are also striving to ensure appropriate *Vigil of Care*. Sometimes women's needs are particularly heightened and their demand for *Care as Vigil and Gift* is great, for example following perinatal loss. Also, when women feel powerless, they may place extra demand on midwives to redress this (Lynch, 2007). Such situations can create significant emotion work for the midwife and striving to meet these needs may become unsustainable. The important thing to recognise here is that human suffering or need may, understandably, contribute to an unbalanced or unsustainable exchange and create emotion work for midwives, some may over-give to compensate or become drained and cope by detaching (Hunter, 2006). Acknowledging this potential imbalance may help us understand what midwives need so they can sustain loving and positive attitudes towards women while maintaining their own wellbeing, such as love for self (Chapter 9) and collegial love and support (Chapter 10). This may avoid midwives using self-protective strategies, such as disengaging, which affect the quality of the mid-wife–mother interaction and women's experiences. Figure 8.2 depicts such exchanges in relation to *gift of care* from the midwife to the woman.

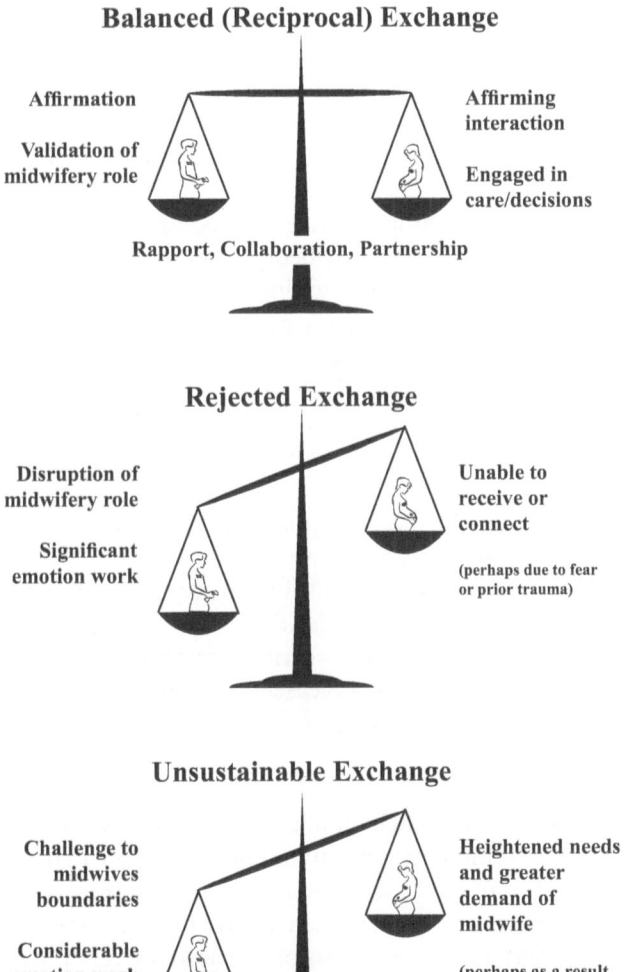

FIGURE 8.2   Exchanges in relation to gift of care from midwives to women.

The nature of gift: the system

Can midwives give too much? Much research suggests yes, perhaps we can and do, with evidence of burnout, trauma, and lack of retention of midwives (Housego, 2023; Hunter et al., 2019; NMC, 2022; Sidhu et al., 2020). Yet arguably this is due not to how much we love or give, but how little we are loved or receive in terms of care and support within our workplaces (Greenstock, 2023; Hunter et al., 2017). See also Chapters 9 and 10. The title "How can we go on caring when nobody here cares about us?" (Reiger & Lane, 2012) resonates with my research that identified how challenging it is for midwives to maintain a compassionate positive approach when the system they work within does not take care of their human needs (Patterson et al., 2019b). When we are not cared for, we might need to disengage, to protect ourselves; this impacts on the quality of midwife–mother interaction and risks birth trauma. A public engagement event showcasing my research findings reflected this with the title "Neglecting midwives gives mothers PTSD" (Beltane Public Engagement network, 2019).

What then is our gift within a system as complex as maternity services. Reiger and Lane (2012) suggest that being a good carer "includes becoming involved in the organisation of care (setting policy, attending meetings), and in supporting junior midwives through kindness, support and encouragement" (p. 135). Importantly, midwives value colleagues showing common sense, taking initiative, and working hard, which makes them feel cared for (Reiger & Lane, 2012). Simple actions such as gifting a listening ear, a cup of tea, moral support, and especially time, can be transformative.

> During a routine third trimester home antenatal visit for a woman whose pregnancy had so far been going very well, my colleague was unable to find a fetal heartbeat. When she called me in tears to tell me, I wanted to support her but wasn't sure how best to. I decided to visit her at home with a home-made chocolate cake. I was a bit worried that cake might be inappropriate or trivial, but my colleague was pleased and found my visit and especially the cake to be very comforting.
>
> *Jane: Midwife, Scotland*

Einion (2023) sees love as a light shining through midwives. The gift of this light can bring clarity and help understanding "something makes sense!" (p. 7). It can lead to inspiration and creative solutions in maternity care, for example, the #hellomynameis…campaign, started in 2013 by Kate Granger MBE (#hellomynameis…, 2024), raised awareness of the need for care providers to introduce themselves and found creative ways of doing this. The clarity from this gift of light can also free individuals and remove any sense of being a burden; it can help us to understand ourselves and each other not only within the midwife–mother relationship, but across multidisciplinary teams.

Forgiveness

A word about forgiveness. When weighing up the costs of gifting care, it can become easy to blame others for our hurt or distress. This can widen the *us* and *them* gap. Yet, as discussed by Godden (2017), forgiveness is the heart of the love ethic. When we take time to reflect lovingly, when we use our emotional intelligence, it becomes possible to stand in others' shoes. This helps us acknowledge the human vulnerability in each of us and to make the choice (love takes choice), to forgive, to engage, and be open to each other. If each member of the maternity care system aims to adopt a loving approach, a benevolent gaze, and unconditional positive regard within whatever role they hold, then creative solutions could be found. This would be a transformative gift to everyone involved and all those who receive care.

Conclusion

This chapter has explored the *how* of maternity care provision within the context of the midwife–mother relationship. It has highlighted that *how* care is provided, whether that be through *Vigil of Care, Care as Gift*, or preferably a combination of both, directly affects the experience of the care provider and recipient, that is the midwife and mother. Whether the experiences are life affirming or traumatic rests largely on the nature of the interaction. The nature of the interaction is influenced by attitude, power, and reciprocity, which in turn depend upon our individual choices. When we choose a loving approach that embodies positive regard and emotional intelligence and are open to forgiveness, it is possible to transform the *how* of maternity care provision.

This is love as gift in midwifery.

References

#hellomynameis… (2024). https://www.hellomynameis.org.uk/

Adib-Hajbaghery, M., & BolandianBafghi, S. (2020). Love in nursing: A concept analysis. *Journal of Caring Sciences*, 9(2), 113–119. https://doi.org/10.34172/JCS.2020.017

Barker, S. (2011). *Midwives' emotional care of women becoming mothers*. Cambridge Scholars Publishing.

Baston, H. (2021). *Midwifery the basics*. Routledge.

Bartunek, J. M. (2019). Contemplation and organization studies: Why contemplative activities are so crucial for our academic lives. *Organization Studies*, 40, 1463–1479.

Bolton, S. C. (2000). Who cares? Offering emotion work as a 'gift' in the nursing labour process. *Journal of Advanced Nursing*, 32(3), 580–586. https://doi.org/10.1046/j.1365-2648.2000.01516.x

Bolton, S. C., Muzio, D., & Boyd-Quinn, C. (2011). Making sense of modern medical careers: The case of the UK's national health service. *Sociology*, 45(4), 682–699.

Beltane Public Engagement Network. (2019). *Cabaret of dangerous ideas – Fringe preview*. https://www.beltanenetwork.org/event/cabaret-of-dangerous-ideas-fringe-preview/

Bryar, R. & Sinclair, M. (2011a). Chapter 1: Signposting future developments in midwifery theory, practice, and research. In R. Bryar, & Sinclair. M. (Eds.), *Theory for midwifery practice* (2nd ed., pp. 3–15). Palgrave Macmillan.

Bryar, R. & Sinclair, M. (2011b). Chapter 3: Midwifery theory development. In R. Bryar, & Sinclair. M. (Eds.), *Theory for midwifery practice* (2nd ed., pp. 59–91). Palgrave Macmillan.

Cambridge Dictionary. (2024). *Definition of care.* https://dictionary.cambridge.org/dictionary/english/care

Coghlan, D. (2023). Contemplating the spirituality of scholarship. *Nursing Philosophy: An International Journal for Healthcare Professionals, 24*(1), e12386. https://doi.org/10.1111/nup.12386

Collins English Dictionary. (2024). *Definition of reciprocity.* https://www.collinsdictionary.com/dictionary/english/reciprocity

Crowther, S., Hunter, B., McAra-Couper, J., Warren, L., Gilkison, A., Hunter, M., Fielder, A., & Kirkham, M. (2016). Sustainability and resilience in midwifery: A discussion paper. *Midwifery, 40*, 40–48. https://doi.org/10.1016/j.midw.2016.06.005

Downe, S., Finlayson, K., Oladapo, O. T., Bonet, M., & Gülmezoglu, A. M. (2018). What matters to women during childbirth: A systematic qualitative review. *PLoS One, 13*(4), e0194906. https://doi.org/10.1371/journal.pone.0194906

Einion, A. (2021). Embracing the power of the 'and'. *Midwifery Matters, Spring, 168*, 36–37.

Einion, A. (2023). Love and light. *The Practising Midwife, 26*(8), 7.

Elmir, R., Pangas, J., Dahlen, H., & Schmied, V. (2017). A meta-ethnographic synthesis of midwives' and nurses' experiences of adverse labour and birth events. *Journal of Clinical Nursing, 26*(23–24), 4184–4200. https://doi.org/10.1111/jocn.13965

El-Nemer, A., Downe, S., & Small, N. (2006). 'She would help me from the heart': an ethnography of Egyptian women in labour. *Social Science & Medicine, 62*(1), 81–92. https://doi.org/10.1016/j.socscimed.2005.05.016

Fox, N. (1993). *Postmodernism, sociology and health.* University of Toronto Press.

Fox, N. (1995). Postmodern perspectives on care: The vigil and the gift. *Critical Social Policy, 15*(44–45), 107–125.

Greenstock, K. (2023). *Flourish: A practical and emotional guidebook to thriving in midwifery.* Pinter & Martin.

Grossman, S., Cooper, Z., Buxton, H., Hendrickson, S., Lewis-O'Connor, A., Stevens, J., Wong, L. Y., & Bonne, S. (2021). Trauma-informed care: Recognizing and resisting re-traumatization in health care. *Trauma Surgery & Acute Care Open, 6*(1), e000815. https://doi.org/10.1136/tsaco-2021-000815

Godden, N.J. (2017). A co-operative inquiry about love using narrative, performative and visual methods. *Qualitative Research, 17*(1), 75–94 https://doi.org/10.1177/1468794116668000

Housego, R. (2023). *MIDIRS Monthly - We need to talk about the midwife mental health crisis.* https://www.midirs.org/latest-news/blog/2023/midirs-monthly-we-need-to-talk-about-the-midwife-mental-health-crisis/

Hunter, B. (2006). The importance of reciprocity in relationships between community-based midwives and mothers. *Midwifery, 22*(4), 308–322. https://doi.org/10.1016/j.midw.2005.11.002

Hunter, B., Fenwick, J., Sidebotham, M., & Henley, J. (2017). *Midwives in the United Kingdom: Levels of burnout, depression, anxiety and stress and associated predictors.*

https://orca.cardiff.ac.uk/id/eprint/125570/1/UK%20WHELM%20accepted%20Manuscript_.pdf

Hunter, B., Fenwick, J., Sidebotham, M., & Henley, J. (2019). Midwives in the United Kingdom: Levels of burnout, depression, anxiety and stress and associated predictors. *Midwifery, 79*, 102526. https://doi.org/10.1016/j.midw.2019.08.008

Kirkham, M. (2010). *The midwife-mother relationship* (2nd ed.). Palgrave.

Kuipers, Y. J. (2022). Exploring the uses of virtues in woman-centred care: A quest, synthesis and reflection. *Nursing Philosophy: An International Journal for Healthcare Professionals, 23*(2), e12380. https://doi.org/10.1111/nup.12380

Leinweber, J., & Rowe, H. J. (2010). The costs of 'being with the woman': Secondary traumatic stress in midwifery. *Midwifery, 26*(1), 76–87. https://doi.org/10.1016/j.midw.2008.04.003

Leinweber, J., Fontein-Kuipers, Y., Karlsdottir, S. I., Ekström-Bergström, A., Nilsson, C., Stramrood, C., & Thomson, G. (2023). Developing a woman-centered, inclusive definition of positive childbirth experiences: A discussion paper. *Birth (Berkeley, Calif.), 50*(2), 362–383. https://doi.org/10.1111/birt.12666

Lynch, K. (2007). Love labour as a distinct and non-commodifiable form or care labour. *The Sociological Review, 55*(3), 550–570.

MacBride-Stewart, S. (2014). Motivations for the 'gift-of-care' in the context of the modernisation of medicine. *Social Theory & Health, 12*(1), 84–104.

Mahon, S. (2016). Love matters. *The Practising Midwife, 19*(3), 42.

McLeod, S. (2024). *Maslow's hierarchy of needs.* Simply Psychology https://www.simplypsychology.org/maslow.html#:~:text=Maslow%27s%20hierarchy%20of%20needs%20is,esteem%2C%20and%20self%2Dactualization

Menage, D., Bailey, E., Lees, S., & Coad, J. (2018). *Women's lived experience of compassionate midwifery.* Doctoral Thesis. Coventry University. Available at: https://www.researchgate.net/publication/385449575_Women's_Lived_Experience_of_Compassionate_Midwifery

Menage, D., Bailey, E., Lees, S., & Coad, J. (2020). Women's lived experience of compassionate midwifery: Human and professional. *Midwifery, 85*, 102662. https://doi.org/10.1016/j.midw.2020.102662

Ménage, D., & Patterson, J. (2020). Compassion as a powerful intervention: How the interactions between women, midwives and maternity services influence women's childbirth experiences and subsequent trauma. *The Practising Midwife, 23*(8). https://www.all4maternity.com/compassion-as-a-powerful-intervention-how-the-interactions-between-women-midwives-and-maternity-services-influence-womens-childbirth-experiences-and-subsequent-trauma?action=genpdf&id=162570

Merriam-Webster. (2024a). *Definition of care.* https://www.merriam-webster.com/dictionary/care

Merriam-Webster. (2024b). *Definition of gift.* https://www.merriam-webster.com/dictionary/gift

Moran, L., Foster, K., & Bayes, S. (2023). What is known about midwives' well-being and resilience? An integrative review of the international literature. *Birth (Berkeley, Calif.), 50*(4), 672–688. https://doi.org/10.1111/birt.12756

Mount, L. (2022). C1 - Stronger together (Original song by Lucy Mount). *Women and Birth: Journal of the Australian College of Midwives, 35*(2), 41. https://doi.org/10.1016/j.wombi.2022.07.115

Nursing and Midwifery Council. (2018). *The code.* https://www.nmc.org.uk/standards/code/read-the-code-online/

Nursing and Midwifery Council. (2022). *NMC register 1st April 2021–31st March 2022.* https://www.nmc.org.uk/globalassets/sitedocuments/data-reports/march-2022/nmc-register-march-2022.pdf

Oakley, A. (1989). William power memorial lecture. Who cares for women? Science versus love in midwifery today. *Midwives Chronicle*, 214–221.

Odorisio, D.M. (2019). *"Contemplating wounds": The spiritual vision of Julian of Norwich.* https://www.ahomeforsoul.com/single-post/2019/04/19/-contemplating-wounds-the-spiritual-vision-of-julian-of-norwich

Patterson, J., Hollins Martin, C.J., & Karatzias, T. (2019a). PTSD post-childbirth: A systematic review of women's and midwives' subjective experiences of care provider interaction. *Journal of Reproductive and Infant Psychology*, *37*(1), 56–83. https://doi.org/10.1080/02646838.2018.1504285

Patterson, J., Hollins Martin, C. J., & Karatzias, T. (2019b). Disempowered midwives and traumatised women: Exploring the parallel processes of care provider interaction that contribute to women developing post traumatic stress disorder (PTSD) post childbirth. *Midwifery*, *76*, 21–35. https://doi.org/10.1016/j.midw.2019.05.010

Peel, N. (2016). Love is a cold climate: midwifery and politics. *Midwifery Matters*, *150*, 8–9.

Perkins, G. (2022). *Conceptualizations of love in social work practice: A naturalistic inquiry.* https://digitalcommons.usm.maine.edu/cgi/viewcontent.cgi?article=1303&context=thinking-matters-symposium

Pulcini, E. (2016). What emotions motivate care? *Emotion Review*, *9*(1), 64–71.

Reed, R., Sharman, R., & Inglis, C. (2017). Women's descriptions of childbirth trauma relating to care provider actions and interactions. *BMC Pregnancy and Childbirth*, *17*(1), 21. https://doi.org/10.1186/s12884-016-1197-0

Reiger, K. & Lane, K. (2012). 'How can we go on caring when nobody here cares about us?' *Australian public maternity units as contested care sites. *Women and Birth*, *26*, 133–137.

Sauro, J. (2015). *Benevolent gazing: The sweet eye of love.* https://www.globalsistersreport.org/spirituality/benevolent-gazing-sweet-eye-love-18771

Sidhu, R., Su, B., Shapiro, K. R., & Stoll, K. (2020). Prevalence of and factors associated with burnout in midwifery: A scoping review. *European Journal of Midwifery*, *4*, 4. https://doi.org/10.18332/ejm/115983

Sorenson, D. S. (2003). Healing traumatizing provider interactions among women through short-term group therapy. *Archives of Psychiatric Nursing*, *17*(6), 259–269. https://doi.org/10.1053/j.apnu.2003.10.002

Sorenson, D.S., & Tschetter, L. (2010). Prevalence of negative birth perception, disaffirmation, perinatal trauma symptoms, and depression among postpartum women. *Perspectives in Psychiatric Care*, *46*(1), 14–25. https://doi.org/10.1111/j.1744-6163.2009.00234.x

Transforming Maternity Care Collaborative. (2024). *Work health and emotional lives of midwives (WHELM).* https://www.transformingmaternity.org.au/work-health-and-emotional-lives-of-midwives-whelm/

Walsh, D. (2011). Chapter 8: Nesting and matrescense. In R. Bryar, & Sinclair. M. (Eds.), *Theory for midwifery practice* (2nd ed., pp. 112–121). Palgrave Macmillan.

PART III
Love in the profession

9

LOVE FOR SELF

Controversies and word games

Kate Greenstock

What is love for self?

There is much to explore about how the concept of self-love has suffered from distortion in the current age. Getting clear on our thoughts and influences is important as we disentangle the verbal and emotional mess we have made of how we see the self.

Loving ourselves, a way of thinking that raises the awareness and value of our individual distinctiveness, characteristics, gifts, and purpose, has been reduced to a commercial catchphrase, exacerbated by the bite-sized power of social media. Wherever you've come across the slogan of *Love yourself*, you've likely been told how important it is to go ahead and do it: to embrace your body as it is; to take pride in who you are and what you've done, even when others don't see it. There is nothing wrong with self-acceptance of course, as long as we are not ignoring a personal struggle that would actually be helpful to address. And it can be all the more necessary when the opposing voices of shame and self-criticism in the world and in our heads are loud, sometimes deafening.

Elizabeth Gilbert (2023) describes self-loathing in our society as a rampant virus. This is confirmed by dramatically escalating numbers of people seeking help for spiralling mental health (House of Commons Library, 2024). The more the virus spreads, the more we require an antidote or a vaccine. This is offered up in the form of self-love. This bite-sized self-love is often rooted in what the Swiss philosopher Rousseau called *amour-propre*: self-love or self-esteem dependent upon the good opinion of others (Rousseau, 2004). While the narrative in social media posts or conversations is about building ourselves *up* as the world (and midwifery) breaks us *down*, we look to other humans for

DOI: 10.4324/9781032645780-13

the affirmation that we are on the right track, interesting to our peers, adventurous, sociable, brave, *good enough* to be acceptable, etc. *Amour de soi*, by contrast, also means *self-love* but is not dependent upon others' affirmation. It is more about staying in touch with our true selves, as Rousseau himself said "If I exercise my reason … if I make good use of my God-given faculties which require no intermediary, I … learn of myself to know [God]" (Rousseau, 1979, p. 307). In other words, I am at peace with myself, and who I was made to be, with no comparisons.

Healthy self-identity as a midwife, a complex story

In my life and work with coaching clients, I have often described this kind of love for self as "coming home to me." The implication here is that we have strayed from *home*, become lost in the deep, dark woods of others' expectations or society's pressures and temptations. We have lost our natural sense of our self. We are so much better off when we can settle into a healthy self-identity. This is a place where, as people and midwives, we can rediscover our individual strengths, values, joys, original motivation, and aliveness in the midst of environments which are increasingly focused on *managing the numbers* rather than human connection and care. Healthy self-identity says, "I know who I am and what's most important to me and I can speak up for it and for others around me." Healthy self-identity says, "I know which elements of this work make me feel alive and I am going to choose roles which match that passion as much as possible." The way we love ourselves begins to be reflected in our emerging knowledge of how we can contribute best to the people around us and to the world.

Vocation: help or hindrance to healthy love for self?

And yet as midwives, we are deeply confused, and sometimes disappointed.

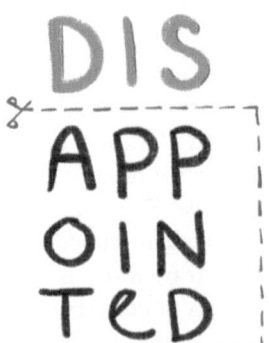

Credit: Jo Bradshaw

We have entered a profession often regarded as a calling or vocation, possibly with a strong sense of purpose, a sense of *appointment* to the work of being *with woman* and enabling the transformational process of pregnancy, birth, and motherhood. Just as those giving birth require courage, so do we, as we sit, as Sheila Kitzinger described it: "on the threshold of life, where intense human emotions – fear, hope, longing, triumph, and incredible physical power – enable a new human being to emerge" (Kitzinger, 2000, p. 164). It's not uncommon for us to be acknowledged in sweet tones by new parents as *angels*, and by the media as *heroes*. While we sometimes choose to buy into these narratives ourselves, both serve ultimately to idealise and depersonalise – leaving less room for us just to be human, imperfect, mistake-making, and tired, living real human lives amidst our acts of so-called heroism. Both make it harder to name the following:

- How deeply emotionally demanding our work can be. In my limited experience, angels and heroes don't appear to experience burnout or compassion fatigue.
- The psychological distress caused by moral injury, the internal battle where we are forced by organisational imperatives to work against our own values.
- The unwritten *rules* or psychological contract at play in the environments we work in. We see leaders and role models regularly going without breaks, staying *above and beyond*, or doing *just another bank shift*, often at a cost to their long-term wellbeing.

The angel and hero narratives presuppose some level of self-sacrifice or selflessness in midwifery. Of course, putting others' needs ahead of our own can be a rich and wonderful way to live. Selflessness may even be part of our sense of direction and purpose in midwifery. Yet the lines start to blur rapidly when we read the distortion in the Cambridge dictionary (2007) definition of vocation as "a type of work that you feel you are suited to doing and *to which you should give all your time and energy*" (my italics). Samantha Batt-Rawden (2021), NHS registrar writing during the Covid-19 pandemic, noted how the image of the hero NHS worker had been appropriated internally "to justify increasingly unsustainable working conditions in the NHS, without care for the needs of those who care for others." It leaves little space, she says, for the hero to be human, and to be asked "how are you?." I would add that it leaves even less space for the midwife to be asked:

"Who are you?" "What are you best at?" "Where do you really thrive?" and "How can you really develop a peaceful and healthy self-regard when the hero narrative is so clearly contradicted by your day-to-day reality and how you feel about yourself at the end of a long shift?"

You can hear the underlying shame in these quotes from early career midwives:

> I didn't speak up for her when it mattered most.
> I went with the flow of the system and what was expected…it's just easier, I guess.

(Personal correspondence, 2021)

It is hard to love ourselves in the midst of such internal contradictions. When we perpetuate dehumanised care, no matter how unwillingly, we become increasingly dehumanised ourselves. We see this pattern emerging over time (Box 9.1).

All of this emphasises the importance of antidotes to self-loathing in midwifery in the form of healthy self-awareness, self-identity, and appreciation (from team and self!).

Love for all aspects of self – dimensions of belonging and psychological safety in the workplace

One of the engines of modern-day medical-industrial style midwifery is fear (Scamell, 2011). Not just the perpetual background fear of something going wrong, but the sensation of *danger* as a result of a lack of psychological safety in teams and leadership behaviours (West, 2021). Fear or a sense of danger keeps us alert and ready for action. It keeps us on the move. And when we experience it persistently, our adrenal system goes into overdrive – a major contributor to burnout.

Team psychological safety, in contrast to fear-driven behaviour, is a shared belief that it's ok to take risks: to suggest a new idea, to tell my boss about my broken heart or my child's illness, to say when something bothers me, to ask when I don't understand, and to be clear and candid when I've made a mistake, all without fearing negative consequences (Edmondson, 2018). How you answer these questions from Amy Edmondson (Edmondson, 2018) will give you a sense of how psychologically safe you feel in your team:

1 If you make a mistake on this team, it is not held against you.
2 Members of this team are able to bring up problems and tough issues.
3 People on this team sometimes accept others for being different.
4 It is safe to take a risk on this team.
5 It isn't difficult to ask other members of this team for help.
6 No one on this team would deliberately act in a way that undermines my efforts.
7 Working with members of this team, my unique skills and talents are valued and utilised.

BOX 9.1   PATTERN OF DEHUMANISED CARE

I am witnessing/involved in episodes of disrespectful care, birth trauma, or coercion as part of my job.

It hurts me because I can't completely protect these families. In "leaving them" vulnerable I am overriding my most strongly held values. In that place, I too am vulnerable.

I am a midwife. It is my role and my pride to be a "guardian" of space, autonomy, and dignity for these women and families.

I want to be the midwife I signed up to be. I want to be "with woman." I should be protecting them and yet I am unable to do so.

I know what is right, and what works for families (and colleagues) but I cannot do it.

I feel some or all of these things: shame, guilt, powerlessness, frustration, overbearing sense of responsibility, lack of motivation, emotional distance from my work and the families, depression, spiritual crisis.

I may experience burnout symptoms such as distancing from the job or from my friends/ family, drinking alcohol every day or to excess, hyper-exercising, hyper-scrolling, becoming excessively busy or over-working as an *avoidance* mechanism, self-harming.

Reproduced with permission from Greenstock (2023)

You can see that so much of this is about encouraging and valuing individuality within a team. And you can imagine how much easier it is to accept and enjoy aspects of yourself when you feel psychologically safe at work, when you feel you can belong, not just *fit in* to the prevailing or dominant culture (Brown, 2021). Indeed, recognising and valuing the gift of *all* aspects of being you, including your personality, preferences, and neurodivergence, is a form of love for self. It involves recognising that those aspects, such as a preference for introversion, observation and gathering thoughts before speaking into a group. This brings enormously diverse gifts to a team or an environment when named, acknowledged, and supported. I am learning, largely through my daughter, that I am a highly sensitive person, which means that I can pick up and guide others through shifts in mood in the room at any time. It supports my work as a coach, facilitator and midwife. Those voices in my younger decades saying I was *too* sensitive, *too* emotional, *too* much, were missing the gift. Part of my expression of love for self has latterly been to choose to work in teams and environments that value my perceptiveness and ability to notice what's needed in the moment. Part of my expression of love for colleagues has been to use that gift with them.

I love the story told of the forest people who began a long march, day after day, when all of a sudden, they stopped walking, sat down and made camp for a couple of days before going further. They explained, when asked, that they needed the time to rest so that their souls could catch up with them.

What if in response to the labour ward lead and her organisational priorities urging *move faster*, *ward her*, we were to say:

No, we have to let our souls catch up.

We, midwife, mother, baby, family, must let our souls catch up. This is part of true care for ourselves and others.

Something sacred has happened. And it can't be rushed.

Love for self by being free to be vulnerable

Closely linked to love for all aspects of ourselves is being brave enough to be vulnerable with each other. I have often mused on what a joy it can be to start a shift with a leader taking 5 minutes not only to welcome newcomers and celebrate small things, but to set a psychologically safe tone for the day or night by being helpfully honest and role-modelling vulnerability about the hours ahead:

This job is tough, especially if for any reason you're feeling less than OK today or didn't sleep well. I'm feeling guilty and sad being here tonight because my child's not well. It's likely that some of you are bringing things with you too. My job tonight is to help you get well fed, watered, and rested. I also want you to feel trusted enough to get on with your work, and to be able to ask questions or tell me if you are worried about anything including mistakes you have made. Remember they are inevitable, and so much more manageable when shared. Please ask for what you need.

Being vulnerable enough to show the cracks in our action-focused armour sets the tone for a kind of emotional holding which makes space for the self in the organisational machine; space for honesty, for needs and questions to appear and to be acceptable, just as in that moment, we remain acceptable.

Vulnerability is a gift, and a practice of love for self. It enables us to ask the hardest question in the midst of our feelings of resentment, overwhelm, fear, or shame:

> What do I need but am afraid to ask for?
> (I need X but worry that if I ask, I will look X, etc.)
>
> *(Brown, 2021, p. 50)*

Brené Brown's research shows how our response to the mismatch between our (often unexpressed) expectations and our reality leads us to be cynical, critical, numb, or semi-engaged. We fear feeling disappointment so deeply that it feels risky even to think through what we need, let alone to say it! So instead, we wear our armour, build our high walls and defences (a trauma exposure response to ongoing disappointment), and press on without looking too hard at what it's costing us.

As Laura van Dernoot Lipsky says in her book *Trauma Stewardship*:

> For many of us, the elaborate architecture we build around our hearts begins to resemble a fortress. We build up our defences, but the trauma keeps on coming. We add a moat, we throw in some crocodiles, we forge more weapons, we build higher and higher walls. Sooner or later, we find ourselves locked in by the very defences we have constructed for our own protection. We will find the key to our liberation only when we accept that what we once did to survive is now destroying us.
>
> *(van Dernoot Lipsky, 2009, pp. 43–44)*

An expression of love for self in this context is choosing to be vulnerable enough to start again; to look for ourselves again amongst the strategic, defensive architecture we have built over time. This is the work I do all the time with coaching clients, and it's amazing to see the work of rediscovery happening, coming *home* again. If you want to explore this further for yourself, go to the exercises in Part 2 of the book *Flourish: a Practical and Emotional Guidebook to Thriving in Midwifery* (Greenstock, 2023). In parallel to this growth in self-awareness, a vital skill is being honed: the art of choosing self-compassion (loving and forgiving and encouraging yourself) over shame. Shame robs us of learning, connection, and a healthy sense of self. Self-compassion restores them all.

Love for self in response to incidents: moving from disgrace to grace

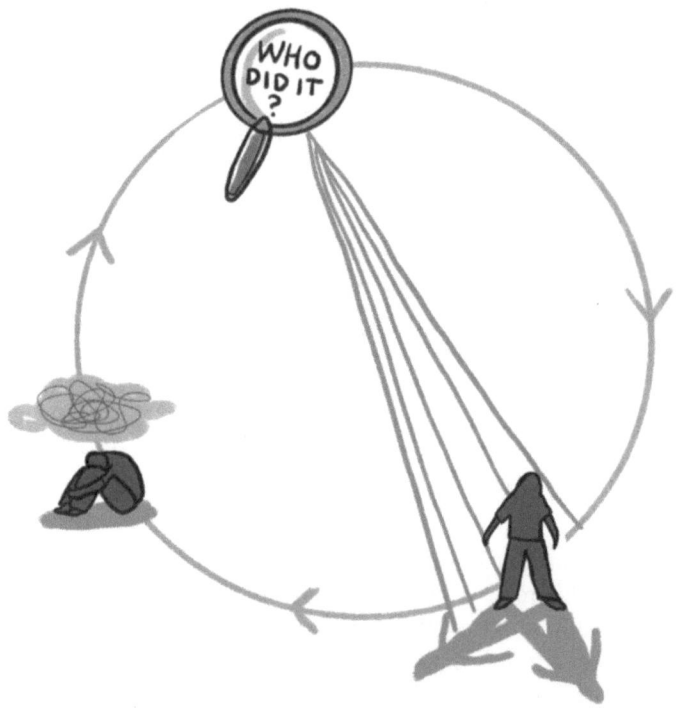

Credit: Jo Bradshaw

Choosing self-compassion over shame is all the more crucial in the intensity of the post-incident moment. We all know that incidents happen in maternity. Complex systemic flaws and failures of teamwork are named repeatedly as the root of mistakes and unsafe practice by government reports (Ockenden, 2022). The knee-jerk reaction in the moment over emphasises the *who done it?* role of the individual, resulting often in self-blame and self-isolation. Substance use is common (Pezaro et al., 2021) as a way of managing the fallout from a near miss or something even more life changing. And we know from the Doctors in Distress charity that medical staff suicides are all too familiar, often in response to the shame fuelled by poorly handled investigations.

It is an act of love for self to seek to understand how our brilliant brains will process and reprocess events. They will often throw up horrifying images sending us into a physiological re-experiencing. Midwife researchers into trauma response Helen Spiby and Pauline Slade (2021) describe this as our attempt to *sort the messy wardrobe* in our brains and store memories into the hippocampus, the appropriate part of the long-term memory that enables us to remember without being *there* anymore. It is also an act of self-love to get the psychological support that we need, from friends, family, and professionals possibly from outside maternity. And finally, the greatest act of self-love, in the midst of a psychological crisis also expressing itself in physiological ways, is to go oh-so-gently. This includes some rest, and some time away from work even though you will hear the old non-evidence-based tropes of "get back in the saddle, it's the best way." It's not, by the way. It's certainly not that simple. Go gently. Listen to these words from Audre Lorde: "We have to study how to be tender with each other until it becomes habit…We can practise being gentle with each other by being gentle with that piece of ourselves [or that memory] that is hardest to hold" (Lorde, 1984, p. 175).

Credit: Jo Bradshaw

Self-care and resilience: confusion and appropriation

Another controversy lies with the notions of resilience and self-care, often explicitly deemed to be the responsibility of the individual midwife to *do her work* on and within herself to stay well. The word resilience has over time developed overtones of the famous wartime recruitment poster with the pointing finger:

Your unit needs YOU (so you'd better find a way to get on with it).

Covid-19 of course accelerated this need for staff to be well. Billie Hunter and Lucie Warren have explored resilience for over a decade. Revisiting the concept in 2022, they note how the word has been "misappropriated by organisational imperatives" as a way of diverting responsibility from the much-needed work of addressing systemic and workforce issues (Hunter & Warren, 2022, p. 10). Psychologist Jan Smith in her book *Nurturing Maternity Staff* suggests that NHS resilience training is "training staff to tolerate a deeply broken system" (Smith, 2021, p. 17).

A dominant narrative fuelled by organisational priorities about becoming a resilient midwife who *bounces back* has also tainted the concept of self-care. We have well-meaningly packaged self-care into the *kale and pedicures* phenomenon (Mathieu, 2021); take exercise, bubble baths, or an occasional gin and tonic or two (with friends of course) to wash away the day or blow off steam, oh and breathe deeply. These soothing *strategies* are presented to us metaphorically gift wrapped or on a freely available app, when what we really need is to work on soothing our systems more deeply, both our own and those of the places we work. The research shows that individual *self-care* strategies may have little impact on reported empathic strain and recovery from trauma exposure and burnout, in comparison with control over the patterns we work and compassionate, high-quality 1-1 and group supervision (Killian, 2008; West, 2021). Our valiant self-care attempts may also get quickly negated when we find ourselves at odds with *self* in so many ways when we hit the squeaky decks at work.

Even mindfulness has been commercialised and co-opted. The Mindfulness-Based Stress Reduction (MBSR) programme over eight weeks has strong validity and shows up in UK National Institute for Health and Clinical Excellence (NICE) guidelines as an evidence-based approach to building and strengthening deeper soothing systems to address clinical diagnoses. Professor Ron Purser's book *McMindfulness* argues that quality mindfulness practice has so much potential to help us raise our collective awareness of what is needed in our workplaces and in the world. He sees it as a travesty that it has become reduced to a convenient *salve* for organisations who would rather classify stress as an individual pathology or maladaptation to the environment and avoid looking too closely at its systemic and structural causes (Purser, 2019). Selling the individual pursuit of mindfulness practice to us as the solution can be seen as a form of extreme gaslighting; it says "you are the problem, look inside yourself" so convincingly that we might well believe it and stop looking outside ourselves at what needs to change.

What is true self care or resilience?

True resilience and radical self-care (radical according to its original meaning of rooted, grounded in self-awareness) is the embodied knowledge that we cannot carry this as individuals, and that the role of the self is intimately connected with the responsibility of the organisation and the system. This might:

1 Start with growing self-awareness, noticing when we are overwhelmed, and practising tiny compassionate shifts in our body and mind which restore us.
2 Generate a love for self mastermove, reaching out for support but also giving it to others. Taking care of ourselves is an act of intention that we will be able to share what we have nurtured.
3 Mobilise us to call out unhealthy or unhelpful behaviours and begin to have brave conversations with ourselves and others as we advocate for a better way, choose to work somewhere different, or on another team, or leave midwifery entirely, for now or forever. There is so much more choice than we are able to see from our frozen state of coping.

Can we call taking care of ourselves a generous act? Possibly, although it is very personal. How much we each need to be available to others can be different. Also, there may be times when we need to continue to act even when our tank is empty. For me, as a Christian, my own experience of faith has shown me the paradox that when I have nothing in the tank, I am often most used/ useful and revived in serving others' needs. In this situation I can in no way claim whatever I do or give as a product of my own resourcefulness, but instead acknowledge it as an act of God's grace and generosity. You might like to reflect on what keeps you going when you have nothing left in the tank.

Truly loving yourself: healthy self-regard in midwifery and in the system

The question lingers: how can we realistically live this out? The first answer to this admittedly complex question is that healthy and honest expectations need to be supported by employers/educators right from the beginning of a midwifery career. Self-love means we can be self-aware enough, even from our time as students, to know how we are highly suited/unsuited to aspects of this work. There is a myth abounding in midwifery that we can all be happy generalists, *fitting in* to a system which requires us to spread thin rather than go deep. Thriving in the system and demonstrating healthy self-regard starts with being honest about where we belong.

The second answer is in establishing and living out healthy workplace boundaries supported by our employers. As midwives, being self-aware can create a clear *Yes* and a clear *No*; it becomes easier to ask for what we need. Identifying role models for the season we are in, whether it is midwifing whilst early mothering, stepping into our first team leader role or being newly qualified; finding an inspiring mentor, one who has walked the path before, makes an enormous difference to feeling less alone as a voice seeking to navigate the system. Healthy boundaries in colleague relationships may involve having courageous conversations, admitting when we feel weak or undermined, asking for feedback or encouragement: most of all naming when something is or is not right so that it can be addressed. The power of healthy boundaries in the mother-midwife psychosocial relationship is often under appreciated. It is tempting, and part of the pervasive public narrative around midwifery, to see ourselves as rescuers, sometimes taking over-responsibility for outcomes and others' lives. It may be a useful reflection for us as midwives to ask ourselves how self-regard for me and deep regard for her might enable a woman to feel and seize responsibility for her own birth and life. A further discussion on boundaries can be found in Chapter 13.

The third answer is in loving our leaders in the hierarchy and loving ourselves as leaders. The hierarchies in organisational (and maternity) systems globally mean that senior leaders describe their roles as lonely (West, 2021). Chapter 11 also highlights this problem.

Many leaders also report suffering from moral injury provoked by the impossible task of caring for staff *and* safety with depleted resources, and having fewer people at work with whom they can be authentic. After two intense years of the Covid-19 crisis, including family illness, one leader reflected with me that not a single colleague had asked her "How are you?." Until our conversation, she hadn't even noticed the absence of the question from colleagues, or from herself.

Leaders with a healthy self-regard are more likely to be able to:

- *Debunk* the myth that good leadership needs a safe distance from the people we lead. Connection and care exist in genuine relationship with others (Walker, 2023; West, 2021).
- Be authentic about personal mental health journeys, role modelling vulnerability.
- Be frank about the psychological challenges of midwifery and the shortcomings of the service.
- Be creative in ways of including diverse voices in exploring ways forward.
- Be free to ask the most important questions:
  - Why do I lead? (i.e. what's the purpose of the leading that I do; what am I trying to shape or create?) (Ledger, 2021, p. 50) and
  - Who do I want to *be* as a leader?

Final reflections

Taking care of ourselves is a generous act; *being cared for* is also a generous act. The person-centred caring we do as midwives cannot happen without those two prerequisites. Interestingly, the biblical phrase "Love your neighbour as yourself" assumes that we know *how* we want to be cared for. And yet often we lack clarity on this very thing. We have much to learn from younger midwives, who tend to have a stronger awareness of boundaries between self and organisation. Yet, therein lies a potential contradiction: an increasingly youthful midwifery workforce may well need support to unpack self-identity and grow in confidence to ask for what's needed. As noted above the hardest question might be:

What do I need but am afraid to ask for?
(I need X but worry that if I ask, I will look X, etc.).

(Brown, 2021, p. 50)

In a maternity system with a feeling of not enough, understandably self-protectedness sets in. This could be understood as a sense of:

What do they need, but I am afraid to give?
(They need X, but I worry that if I give it [in the way they need it] I will suffer in X ways)

There is an abundant overspill of love and care that flows from deeply knowing ourselves, accepting and receiving love. Bold collective conversations about creating and sustaining loving environments in maternity are imperative if we are to create and sustain self-and (m)other-loving midwives.

References

Batt-Rawden, S. (2021, May 1). We need to stop calling NHS staff heroes – for a very important reason. *The Independent.* https://www.independent.co.uk/voices/nhs-covid-stress-burnout-heroes-b1840683.html

Brown, B. (2021). *Atlas of the heart: Mapping meaningful connection and the language of human experience.* Ebury Publishing.

Cambridge Essential English dictionary. (2007). 10th Ed. Cambridge University Press.

Edmondson, A. (2018). *The fearless organization: Creating psychological safety in the workplace for learning, innovation, and growth.* John Wiley & Sons.

Gilbert, E. (2023). *Welcome to letters of love.* https://elizabethgilbert.substack.com/p/welcome-to-letters-from-love

Greenstock, K. (2023). *Flourish: A Practical and Emotional Guidebook to Thriving in Midwifery.* Pinter & Martin.

Hunter, B., & Warren, L. (2022). Revisiting Resilience. *The Practising Midwife, 25,* 9–13.

House of Commons Library. (2024). *Mental Health Statistics: prevalence, services and funding in England.* https://researchbriefings.files.parliament.uk/documents/SN06988/SN06988.pdf

Killian, K. D. (2008). Helping till it hurts? A multimethod study of compassion fatigue, burnout, and self-care in clinicians working with trauma survivors. *Traumatology, 14*(2), 32–44. http://dx.doi.org/10.1177/1534765608319083

Kitzinger, S. (2000). *Rediscovering Birth.* Little Brown.

Ledger, K. (2021). Person Centred and Compassionate Leadership. In: J. Smith. *Nurturing Maternity Staff: How to Tackle Trauma, Stress and Burnout to Create a Positive Working Culture in the NHS* (pp. 44–60). Pinter & Martin.

Lorde, A. (1984). *Sister Outsider: Essays and Speeches*. The Crossing Press.

Mathieu, F. (2021). *Beyond Kale and Pedicures: Can we beat Burnout & Compassion Fatigue?* https://www.tendacademy.ca/beyond-kale-and-pedicures/

Ockenden, D. (2022). *Final report of the Ockenden review. Findings, conclusions and essential actions from the independent review of maternity services at the Shrewsbury and Telford Hospital NHS Trust.* Department of Health and Social Care. https://www.gov.uk/government/publications/final-report-of-the-ockenden-review

Personal correspondence. (2021). With newly qualified midwives.

Pezaro, S., Maher, K., Bailey, E., & Pearce, G. (2021). Problematic substance use: An assessment of workplace implications in midwifery. *Occupational medicine (Oxford, England)*, *71*(9), 460–466. https://doi.org/10.1093/occmed/kqab127

Purser, R. (2019). *McMindfulness: How Mindfulness Became the New Capitalist Spirituality*. Repeater books.

Rousseau, J. J. (2004). *Discourse on the origin of inequality*. Dover Publications.

Rousseau, J. J. (1979). *Emile or On Education. Introduction, translation and notes by Allan Bloom*. Basic Books.

Scamell, M. (2011). The swan effect in midwifery talk and practice: a tension between normality and the language of risk. *Sociology of Health & Illness*, *33*(7), 987–1001. https://doi.org/10.1111/j.1467-9566.2011.01366.x

Slade, P., & Spiby, H. (2021, October 5). *Together We Can Care for Each Other*. Online RCM Conference.

Smith, J. (2021). *Nurturing Maternity Staff: How to Tackle Trauma, Stress and Burnout to Create a Positive Working Culture in the NHS*. Pinter & Martin.

van Dernoot Lipsky, L., & Burk, C. (2009). *Trauma Stewardship: An Everyday Guide to caring for Self While Caring for Others*. Berrett-Koehler.

Walker, E. (2023). *Henri Nouwen on leadership*. https://gracetruth.blog/2023/08/30/henri-nouwen-on-leadership-by-ed-walker/

West, M. (2021). *Compassionate Leadership: Sustaining Wisdom, Humanity and Presence in Health and Social Care*. The Swirling Leaf Press.

10

LOVE AND COLLEAGUES

Sustaining wellbeing in the workplace through social connections

Sheena Byrom and Anna Byrom

Introduction

Throughout this book, so far, you have learnt why love counts during child-bearing, birth, and beyond, enabling quality midwifery care. In this chapter, you will consider the social nature of love and how love can transform our lives, across our workplace relationships and cultures. The impact of our working environments, team dynamics, and organisational culture will be presented alongside a meaningful map charting ways to foster loving connections and community across our maternity and perinatal services. This chapter begins with a focused consideration of social love: love as social connection. We then consider the global and national position of midwifery, challenges within working environments, and explore solutions for sustaining wellbeing at work and positively influencing the culture in maternity services.

Social love: constructs and concepts of community connection

From the moment of our conception, we function in relation to our environment, and as human beings, from our birth, we seek connection through our relationships with our parents, family, and wider communities. Brene Brown believes that "love, belonging, connection, and joy are irreducible needs for all of us. We can't give people what we don't have. We have to live love to give love" (Brown, 2019).

Across each chapter of this book, you have explored the ways in which love matters to human flourishing. Here, we examine our social need to connect in our workplace relationships, environments, and organisational cultures.

DOI: 10.4324/9781032645780-14

Understanding the social constructs of love helps us to unpack the meaning of loving relationships across our working lives.

Love has been well documented across the arts with copious volumes of literature, paintings, and modern media dedicated to its exploration. Within the scientific community there have been moves to understand the physiology of love, attributed to our hormonal responses and the influence of oxytocin, which is sometimes called the *love hormone*. Advancements across psychology have helped to identify psychological perceptions of love tied to the emotional realm revealed across thoughts, feelings, and behaviours. Chapter 1 provides greater insight into the different theories of love.

Based on the work of sociologists (Durkheim, 1893; Sorokin, 1954; Weber, 1922), we propose love as a moral social duty to each other in our work as maternity healthcare professionals and workers; love is a force to transform working environments and cultures.

Every single human being is worthy of being loved as a *brother* (community member) based on the universality of human suffering (Weber, 1922).

Contemporary sociologists have linked our most personal and intimate feelings to our social nature, conveying how the transformational potential of love and intimacy promotes vast social change (Bauman, 2003; Beck & Beck-Gernsheim, 1995; Illouz, 2012, 2018; Luhmann, 1986). In their edited book, Cataldo and Iorio (2022) extend the debate on social love and its potential for transformative force in a time of ongoing social crises and concern. Table 10.1 describes the four dimensions of social love, presented across the chapters of their book and summarised succinctly by Montagna (2023).

For midwives and maternity workers, these dimensions can be utilised when caring for women, families, and our colleagues, for example, taking action to provide support or care even when it isn't expected, and being open and

TABLE 10.1 Four dimensions of social love adapted from Cataldo and Iorio (2022) and Montagna's (2023) summary

Overabounding	*Care*	*Universalism*	*Recognition*
Exceeding shared expectations for care and connection by doing more than the situation requires, so more than just duty. Love is an action, practical and more than just sensitivity and feeling.	How we open ourselves to others and the world. Two fundamental features: practical care alongside attention and empathy.	Social love is not only for those people in our own social circle or those similar to us.	The notion that social love is a bond that enhances differences rather than suppressing them allowing people the right to be themselves.

self-aware with our beliefs and predetermined prejudices to connect with others, especially those who are different to us, striving to be welcoming and authentic. The potential impact from acts of kindness is immense. Consider the last time someone was kind to you, helping you or sending a comforting message. From the moment of birth our brains are biologically wired to respond to the care and kindness from others (Gilbert, 2009).

Love can be understood as a social force with the potential to build a sense of community, care, and connection in any context, including throughout our workplaces. Our workplaces are social environments where relationships can either flourish or be diminished. Relational-Cultural Theory (Baker Miller, 1976) serves as a framework that conceptualises the idea that individuals require social connections with others, through an interactive process, in order to flourish, and that cultural practices of categorising individuals can influence their relationships. Baker-Miller's framework contends that the workplace can be a hostile environment where the qualities of nurturing and kindness can be viewed as weaknesses. However, viewed through the lens of social interaction theory, workplace civility, courteous and polite behaviours that are used in respectful interactions are a foundational component of building social connections (Andersson & Pearson, 1999). A more recent approach was extended by the work of Di Fabio and Gori (2016) who introduced the concept of relational civility (RC) that is characterised by respect and concern for oneself and others. Building on RC, Di Fabio and Duradoni (2019) have developed their workplace relational civility (WRC), a more comprehensive framework and scale that helps to capture the relational needs of people in the workplace in relation to civility.

Setting the scene: disappearing midwives

Issues associated with lack of staffing in midwifery have been raised in Chapters 6 and 7; this is a real issue in the context of today's maternity care, especially in light of the world shortage of midwives (Nove et al., 2021). We explore some of the reasons midwives appear to be *disappearing* and how we can meaningfully retain those who stay. Whilst midwifery may be seen by many as a worthwhile *calling*, with midwives held in high regard, there is a long and detailed history of the oppression and vilification of midwives (Donnison, 1988). Gender, race, and class-based marginalisation of the profession is a global concern, with a struggle for autonomy, particularly in a patriarchal, colonial system, being an ongoing challenge for midwives (Ashley et al., 2022). This position may influence the recruitment of midwives globally and nationally. In the United Kingdom, there is an ongoing decline in the number of applications to study midwifery (Royal College of Midwives [RCM], 2023).

Whilst there is an increasing urgency to recruit more midwives and to make midwifery an attractive and satisfying career, the focus on the retention of those midwives currently in practice is of critical importance (Cull et al., 2020;

Moncrieff et al., 2023). Many midwives are quitting the profession, reporting that they feel underappreciated, burnt out, disillusioned, and unable to give quality care (Albendín-García et al., 2021; Cramer & Hunter, 2019; Harvie et al., 2019; Hunter et al., 2019; Mohammad et al., 2020). It is a vicious circle. As midwives continue to leave, the ones who remain are further burdened, feeling the consequences of reduced numbers available to work, which ultimately leads to more stress, exhaustion, and poor psychological health.

So, why are midwives leaving? Most midwives enter the profession to make a difference to society, contribute to women's reproductive health, to nurture, and to care. Gaining a place to study midwifery, and then negotiating an academic degree, as well as learning clinical skills in the workplace, is no mean feat. Qualified midwives have invariably endured many challenges as well as opportunities during their years of training and practising. When their expectations are firmly fixed on the desire to provide woman-centred care and the opposite is experienced, midwives report feeling disillusioned and then leave (Cramer & Hunter, 2019; Hunter et al., 2019). In a recent study, midwives reported the lack of ability to provide quality care as the top reason why they intended to leave, along with insufficient staff, impact on mental health, burnout, and high workload (Moncrieff et al., 2023). In her book on nurturing maternity staff, Dr Jan Smith (2021) identifies the experience of moral distress and moral injury as being a potential contributor to the exodus of midwives. In addition, the unyielding medicalisation of childbirth is impacting on midwives' wellbeing (Mayra et al., 2023), with some suffering post-traumatic stress disorder symptoms following exposure to traumatic perinatal events (Sheen et al., 2015). These working conditions and experiences can and do influence the behaviour of staff and overall culture within maternity workspaces (Mayra et al., 2023).

Incivility and bullying

Alongside this challenging landscape is the reporting of bullying in midwifery (Capper et al., 2020; Gillen et al., 2008; Winter, 2023). In a recently published report dedicated to this topic, midwives shared deeply traumatic accounts of toxic cultures where bullying by individuals and groups was a common denominator and sometimes the cause of midwives leaving the profession (Hughes, 2023). Bullying is both a consequence and symptom of negative culture and poor leadership (Byrom, 2022) and can be interprofessional and at any level or grade. Whilst the literature cited here focuses on the bullying of midwives and student midwives, intimidating behaviour is passed on, revealed here by a doctor on a social media platform (Tam, 2024):

I've also been bullied by midwives when I was a med student. Now I'm terrified of them and my next rotation is O&G. And I DEFINITELY see a big difference with how they treat male vs female doctors.

This phenomenon has been highlighted previously. A forum theatre company who perform nationally to support the work of midwives delivered a scenario as part of their repertoire called *Swimming in Concrete* (Progress Theatre, n.d.). The scene portrays bullying in maternity services using an example from the labour ward, from various perspectives. It is a cascade effect. The shift coordinator feels bullied by the midwifery manager and in turn bullies the midwives on duty. They respond with similar behaviours to the junior doctor, who then mirrors the behaviour towards the student midwife. It is a vicious circle of learned toxic behaviour feeding a culture of disrespect and mistrust. Incivility and unkindness in healthcare is a common but unacceptable phenomenon which can lead to psychologically unsafe working environments for employees and potentially for those using them (Patterson et al., 2019).

In England, there has been a succession of maternity service investigations (Kirkup, 2015, 2022; Ockenden, 2022), where devastating harm was incurred by mothers and babies. Threaded throughout each report is the acknowledgement of poor interprofessional relationships and a lack of compassion shown to families. We need to find different ways of exploring these problems in maternity care that will focus on reducing undermining and negative cultures because they are harming the care women and families receive (Crowther et al., 2019). But what makes individual maternity care workers feel compelled to be disrespectful and detached from human connection in this way? External and internal pressures as described above, where midwives and doctors feel disempowered and uncared for, can lead to a lack of meaning and compassion between staff and those they serve (Patterson et al., 2019).

Fear can also contribute to toxic working environments. When maternity care systems exist within a culture of blame and recrimination, routine defensive practices become commonplace and childbirth is reduced to a conveyor belt system where efficiency and risk management are prioritised over personalised care (Crowther et al., 2019). Midwives and doctors work in trepidation, fearful of making a mistake or omission, which may lead to recrimination and litigation. Any organisation fostering a blame culture is creating a potentially psychologically and clinically unsafe environment where *covering your back* and mistrust become the norm. Incivility and disrespect are often a symptom of this workplace culture where colleagues become unkind to each other, unhelpfully forming cliques. This leads to a *us* and *them* culture which leads to bullying and may predispose to fear and a reluctance to report concerns, leading to unsafe practices adversely affecting women, newborns, and families (Mayra et al., 2023).

Us and *them* culture refers to a social or organisational dynamic where there is a clear divide between two groups, often leading to feelings of opposition, mistrust, or conflict. This division can occur in various settings, such as workplaces, communities, or larger societal groups, and is typically characterised by an *in-group* (the *us*) and an *out-group* (the *them*). In maternity services, conflicts can occur between night and day staff, hospital and community teams, different races, colours or religions, and between midwives and doctors. The professional tensions between midwives and doctors, where hierarchical dynamics exist, is well documented (Donnison, 1988; Leap & Hunter, 2014; Lephard, 2024; Teijlingen, 2018). The dominant medical model, with a focus on pathology, often conflicts with the midwifery model in which the focus is on physiology. When one group holds more power, authority, or privilege, feelings of resentment or injustice can manifest in the less powerful group. This power imbalance can reinforce the division and make it more difficult to bridge the gap. Mutually respectful relationships, which enable open communication and dialogue between groups and enhance understanding, is the solution (as also discussed in Chapter 13). Strategies to encourage collaboration, such as joint education and restorative sessions, are helpful in encouraging multi-professional relationships, examples of which are outlined in the following sections.

Transforming the workplace culture: what can we do?

There is a global drive to promote compassionate care as a fundamental component of quality health services (West, 2021; Youngson, 2012) and midwifery and maternity care (Byrom, 2022; Byrom & Downe, 2015; Crowther et al., 2019; Greenstock, 2023; Hall, 2013; Krausé et al., 2020; Menage et al., 2020; Smith, 2021; Uvnäs-Moberg; 2015). We believe this compassion should be extended to our colleagues too. The culture of any health service workplace depends on the positive regard and mutual respect employees have for each other. In fact, positive, supportive relationships with work colleagues can make the difference between staying in the midwifery profession and leaving it:

> I go to work each day because I love the people that I work with…It's a huge reason why I stay.
>
> *(Bloxsome et al., 2020, p. 213)*

West (2021) maintains that we are all responsible for the culture in our workplace across every ward, department, and speciality. What we say, how we say it, and how we show up every day, matters. Having said that, each member of the maternity team needs to be supported and nurtured and to feel valued and psychologically safe. Mayra et al. (2023) stress the importance of organisations creating compassionate working environments where midwives are listened to, and attention is paid to their needs. There are useful examples from healthcare organisations where strategic approaches to fostering a compassionate, inclusive and collaborative ethos have positively influenced the workplace culture (NHS Leadership Academy, 2022; West, 2021). For individual inspiration and encouragement, Smith (2021) and Greenstock (2023) have crafted exquisite books specifically for maternity staff and midwives. Learning from others is a great way to start. Being open to ideas and exploring ways of doing things differently can be helpful, and the podcast series from the NHS Leadership Academy (2022) is accessible and free!

> A physical hug from those that truly understand a situation can make so much difference. It can say so much without words. I'd had a tough shift and felt emotional. A concerned and caring arm around my shoulder steered me to a quiet corner and didn't ask for me to explain. She just gave me a hug and told me I was a brilliant midwife. I felt so lucky to be part of a team and profession full of amazing people, capable of phenomenal things. After a night of feeling like I was working in an unsafe setting due to poor staffing and lack of support available, I felt safe in her arms. What we do for women and birthing people, we can do for each other.
>
> *Midwife – anonymous*

Compassion is love in action

Skilled, heartfelt midwifery practice is the term coined by Dr Claire Feeley in her PhD study exploring the experiences of midwives who facilitated *alternative physiological births* within their practice. Feeley (2023) found that participants "demonstrated high levels of empathy and compassion" (p. 98) for those they served when hearing their accounts of previous trauma or distress. The midwives shared the fact that they *loved* the women they cared for, and they *loved* birth, revealing their passion for their work. For these situations to manifest successfully, midwives expressed the need for empathy and compassion to be afforded them too, in respectful, encouraging working environments where they were supported and nurtured by their peers and managers (Feeley, 2023). Midwives need love. Brene Brown (2019) confirms this notion stating, "we need love wherever there are humans – that means at work too."

Compassion is viewed as a manifestation of love and by West (2021, p. 1) as a "universal human value." In his book on compassionate leadership in health and social care, West (2021) suggests that compassion creates a sense of belonging that ripples out like a chain reaction. When we experience loving, kind, or compassionate behaviours from others, our colleagues, or family members, it often brings joy, relief, or comfort. This immediate positive emotion can improve our mood and outlook, and we are more likely to act kindly and compassionately towards others (Gilbert, 2009; West, 2021; Youngson, 2015). Experiencing kindness can increase a person's empathy, making them more attuned to the needs of others and more likely to offer help or support in the future (Smith, 2021). As kindness spreads, it can transform the atmosphere on a shift, within a department and even an organisation (Byrom, 2022). A culture of kindness and compassion fosters cooperation, reduces conflicts, and strengthens social bonds

(West, 2021). However, leadership plays a crucial part by role modelling behaviours for others to follow.

West (2021) describes four elements of compassionate leadership as attending, understanding, empathising, and helping. This guides healthcare workers in understanding the fundamentals of this powerful, authentic leadership style. See Table 10.2. Compassionate leadership offers a meaningful framework to use with each other and with colleagues within our workplace communities.

Whilst reflecting on world events in 2019 and the fear she was feeling, Brene Brown shared her decision to *double down* on love and renewed her commitment to living by a *love ethic* (Brown, 2019). As she prepared her list of actions to take for this, Brown committed to nurture and protect love and kindness in herself and others. The eight changes she proposes are enlightening and inspiring and focus mainly on love, joy, and gratitude, to counteract the *dominant*

TABLE 10.2 Compassionate care for colleagues including practical suggestions for everyday use

Compassionate care for colleagues principles	*Attending*	*Understanding*	*Empathising*	*Helping*
Summary	Giving time and listening with fascination to your colleague.	Checking understanding from your colleagues' point of view.	Sharing feelings, putting yourself in your colleagues' shoes.	Offering practical support to help your colleague.
Examples	Responding to colleagues, giving time to each other. Team check-ins at the beginning or end of the shift. Meaningful supervision and support. Health and wellbeing sessions.	Reflecting back and asking questions. Restorative supervision.	Consideration of people's feelings. Non-judgemental check-ins. Chance to explore team emotions and perspectives.	Offer care – comfort and support. Consider practical solutions and help make a meaningful plan.

paradigm. We can only know love if we let go of power and domination. This certainly resonates with our experience as midwives. During our careers, we have experienced both positive and negative behaviours from colleagues. We have both been subjected to extensive bullying, and disrespectful attitudes from colleagues. Thankfully, we have also experienced positive influences from managers and peers who have nurtured and supported us at every level. It was not always easy to focus on *joy*, for example, during a difficult time, or to feel gratitude when the chips were down. By really trying to concentrate on what we *could* do, and reconnecting with our purpose as midwives and to our values, we were able to succeed. The relinquishing of any perceived power and control that comes with being a midwife was and is important to us both; the woman is always the central focus, and we are her professional servant (Cronk, 2000). The philosophy of woman or person-centred care is integral to how we practise, and as we gained promotion within our individual midwifery careers in leadership and education, the underpinning impetus of our actions remained the same.

Working alongside positive role models who genuinely cared, who led by example and moulded our practice made us aware of strategies to sustain midwifery practice and promote wellbeing. Our interest in encouraging loving relationships has given us the impetus to share what we know, during our lives and our work.

The loving impact

When we consider love in maternity care, we immediately think of the importance of the hormone oxytocin and how we can optimise its production. Oxytocin, sometimes known as the love hormone, supports optimal reproduction, childbirth, mother–infant connection and lactation. In addition to encouraging social connection and lowering tension and anxiety, oxytocin also promotes calmness and relaxation (Buckley & Uvnäs-Moberg, 2019). With this knowledge, it seems reasonable to suggest that oxytocin is something we all need in our work as midwives and maternity workers. If compassion and love form the basis of all our actions, therefore encouraging the secretion of oxytocin, we could feel the benefits of this when providing care.

When our working environment is pressured and challenging and we feel stressed, cortisol is secreted, and oxytocin production is dampened. Understanding this, and utilising strategies to counteract or prevent this physiological response is useful in promoting wellbeing at work. Small acts of kindness, symbols of love, positively influence staff and the organisations they work in. When individuals feel valued and experience kindness from others, it may lead them to feel joy, gratitude, and inspiration which in turn can enhance individual wellbeing (Greenstock, 2023; Smith, 2021; West, 2021).

In 2024, we conducted an online survey using social media channels, inviting midwives and maternity workers to explore experiences from practice. We asked:

We are writing a book chapter on workplace culture and the need for compassion, kindness and respect to be given to and between maternity workers as well as those they care for. We're focusing on LOVE in midwifery and maternity care, how love can be shared between colleagues. Would you kindly share your thoughts?

Fifty-seven responses were received, the majority from midwives and student midwives. We asked participants if they had ever been bullied and, sadly, 96.5% had. Then we invited them to share a time when they felt cared for or supported lovingly and nurtured by colleagues, and if so, what did the person do? This is where we felt encouraged by most of the responses, which included:

For me, love is the heart of all human behaviour. It's the most powerful human emotion. We fight for the things we love; love is what makes us. So, bringing love into the core of everything we do, you would think midwifery would be filled with love, given we are nurturing the love hormone! We have lost this love, not because we don't have it, it's buried inside layers of institutional fear, disappointment, apathy, covering up our love for one another. I know it's there deep down, it's how we get back to it, find the love for one another. Midwife – anonymous

When I first started 8 years ago, I will never forget a senior midwife taking the time to make sure I ate and had a brew and just listened when all I wanted to do was quit after a particularly bad day. Her kindness and words made all the difference, so much so I asked her to be a significant part in my wedding day (she's also a registrar) and she married me and my husband. Midwife – anonymous

There is a midwife I work with who is effortlessly cheerful, as in, it's not plastering the cracks, she just is that way. Even when things are tough, she always makes sure that she takes the time to speak to you and support you if she can. She never, ever gets into conversations about other people (unless it's positive!) so you know she won't share things behind your back. She will let you have a moan and she won't make you feel like what you're going through doesn't matter, but she has this way of being positive that makes it hard not to feel great around her. Midwife – anonymous.

Since it is genuine and not forced it never feels patronising. Working with her always makes me feel better because I know no matter how tough the shift is she will still be smiling; she will still be calm, and we will get through it together. She makes me feel more positive about everything, just by being around her. It makes me feel like it can be true that staffing is rubbish, and some days are hard and sometimes I don't want to be at work but also at the same time there can be positivity too. They are not mutually exclusive, and I think that's really important. It's not about relentless positivity, there is a balance and people being able to vent and talk about their frustrations is important too. Midwife – anonymous.

The above words from midwives show that love and compassion to others can take very little time, and yet make an enormous difference to individuals, teams, departments, and organisations.

Authenticity and meaning

In his book *Time to Care*, Robin Youngson (2012) captured the need to focus on strengthening working relationships as part of the solution to building happy and fulfilling practice, wellbeing at work, and resilience. The same author, Youngson (2015), reflected on how his behaviour as an obstetric anaesthetist influenced work–place relationships either negatively or positively, and through a shift in his own attitude following his daughter's serious accident, he improved the relationships he had with labour ward midwives and ultimately, the experience of those in his care. Youngson shared an idea that can help to encourage positive collaborative working and promote a supportive workplace culture (Youngson, 2014). The ACT (with compassion) mnemonic, encourages healthcare workers to Appreciate, Commend, and Teach in working environments by authentically acknowledging each other's contributions. This is mobilised by firstly *Appreciation* of any action we witness at work that we feel has made a positive difference to care given. Then *Commending* the person and action to others, publicly informing work colleagues of what we have witnessed. Inviting the celebrated colleague to then *Teach* others, if appropriate, closes the circle and supports the sharing of good practice. The key to this action is that the feedback must be meaningful and specific. Using ACT is in sharp contrast to the blame and shame culture that often exists in healthcare services. The following experience of a student midwife shows how this kind of feedback can make a difference.

Jane, a qualified midwife, was in the postnatal area at work when she overheard a student midwife, Louise, giving a mother discharge information at the bed side, behind the bed screens. Jane was impressed with Louise's communication style and use of jargon-free language. When Louise finished and came out from behind the screens, Jane commended Louise and told her exactly why she was impressed with her practice (Appreciate). Louise was surprised and embarrassed at the time, but later felt proud that she had received such positive feedback. Jane went to the desk where several staff members were present and she shared what she had just witnessed (Commending). Jane then encouraged other students and midwives to listen to Louise in the future, so that they too could learn how to meaningfully share information to those in their care (Teaching). Louise told one of us this story, informing us that it was one of the highlights of her midwifery training.

Being proactively supportive of work colleagues in this way can help to promote and sustain a loving working environment where staff feel valued and important. This action supports the building of relationships and caring connections.

Engendering love in practice – shifting the culture

In her book on nurturing maternity staff, Jan Smith (2021) encourages the practice of *reaching in* to others as a way of caring and supporting. We often ask our colleagues in passing how they are, without stopping to really hear. In addition, colleagues may be struggling and not feeling able to respond. Taking time to stop and to ask, "How are you?" in a meaningful way and waiting for an answer can be helpful (Smith, 2021). Smith shares examples of small actions that may help team members to feel valued, such as checking in via text message, making a colleague a drink and giving positive feedback. These small acts create virtuous circles of loving connection and support, if the receiver replicates the actions to others.

> Being interested in others – not wanting to know the in/outs but listening when someone says something has happened in their own lives. Checking in on them – not always by seeing them but a little message via WhatsApp or a text. Midwife – anonymous

It is not always easy. Sometimes we feel overwhelmed ourselves and unable to consider the problems others are facing. When this happens, Jan Smith suggests we practise ACT – yes the same mnemonic as above, but with different meaning – Acceptance and Commitment Therapy. This means learning to acknowledge and accept the emotion we are feeling (e.g., anger, frustration, fear) whilst making a commitment to act in a manner consistent to our values (Smith, 2021). In her book, Smith suggests ways of practising this as it may not be easy to achieve at first. LOVE – Living Our Values Everyday– remembering who we are and what matters to us can support our personal wellbeing and fulfilment. Love makes a difference (Smith, 2021).

The future

Love, understood as a powerful social force, has the potential to transform work environments, fostering a sense of community, care, and mutual respect.

This chapter has explored the significant challenges facing midwives, from the global shortage of practitioners to the toxic cultures of bullying and incivility that pervade many healthcare settings. These challenges undermine the wellbeing of healthcare workers and compromise the quality of care provided to women and their families.

The concept of social love, grounded in both historical and contemporary sociological thought, offers a pathway to improving workplace cultures. By embracing relational–cultural theories and practices, midwives and maternity care professionals can begin to work lovingly, rebuilding trust and compassion within their teams. This shift requires a collective effort from all members of the healthcare community, including leadership, to model and promote behaviours that prioritise empathy, understanding, and practical support.

Transforming workplace culture in maternity services is not just about addressing the symptoms of dysfunction, such as burnout and bullying, but about fostering a deep, systemic change that aligns with the core values of midwifery: compassion, respect, and a commitment to the wellbeing of both caregivers and those they serve. By cultivating a culture of love in action, we can create work environments where midwives and other healthcare professionals feel valued, supported, and inspired to stay in their roles, ultimately leading to better outcomes for everyone involved.

As we move forward, it is crucial to recognise that the way we treat each other in our professional lives matters just as much as the care we provide. A compassionate, loving workplace culture not only enhances job satisfaction and retention but also directly contributes to the quality of care delivered. Through commitment to these principles, we can ensure that maternity and perinatal services are places where both professionals and patients can thrive.

References

Albendín-García, L., Suleiman-Martos, N., Cañadas-De la Fuente, G. A., Ramírez-Baena, L., Gómez-Urquiza, J. L., & De la Fuente-Solana, E. I. (2021). Prevalence, related factors, and levels of burnout among midwives: A systematic review. *Journal of Midwifery & Women's Health, 66*(1), 24–44. https://doi.org/10.1111/jmwh.13186

Andersson, L. M., & Pearson, C. M. (1999). Tit for tat? The spiraling effect of incivility in the workplace. *Academy of Management Review, 24*(3), 452–471. https://doi.org/10.5465/amr.2000.3312921

Ashley, R., Goodarzi, B., Horn, A., de Klerk, H., Ku, S. E., Marcus, J. K., Mayra, K., Mohamied, F., Nayiga, H., Sharma, P., Udho, S., Vijber, M. R., & van der Waal, R. (2022). A call for critical midwifery studies: Confronting systemic injustice in sexual, reproductive, maternal, and newborn care: Critical Midwifery Collective Writing Group. *Birth (Berkeley, Calif.), 49*(3), 355–359. https://doi.org/10.1111/birt.12661

Baker Miller, J. (1976). *Toward a new psychology of women*. Beacon Press

Bauman, Z. (2003). *Liquid love: On the frailty of human bonds*. Polity Press.

Beck, U., & Beck-Gernsheim, E. (1995). *The normal chaos of love*. Polity Press.

Bloxsome, D., Bayes, S., & Ireson, D. (2020). "I love being a midwife; it's who I am": A Glaserian Grounded Theory Study of why midwives stay in midwifery. *Journal of Clinical Nursing, 29*(1–2), 208–220. https://doi.org/10.1111/jocn.15078

Brown, B. (2019, October 9). *Doubling down on love.* https://brenebrown.com/articles/2019/10/09/doubling-down-on-love/

Buckley, S. & Uvnäs-Moberg, K. (2019). Nature and consequences of oxytocin and other neuro-hormones during the perinatal period. In S. Downe & S. Byrom (Eds.), *Squaring the circle: Normal birth research, theory and practice in a technological age* (pp. 19–31). Pinter and Martin.

Byrom, S. & Downe, S. (2015). T*he roar behind the silence: Why kindness, warmth, compassion and respect matter in maternity care.* Pinter and Martin.

Byrom, S. (2022). Nurturing humanity in Midwifery: compassionate mindful leadership. In S. Crowther & L. Davies (Eds.), *Mindfulness in the birth sphere: Practice for pre-conception to the critical 1000 days and beyond* (pp. 249–265). Routledge.

Capper, T., Muurlink, O., & Williamson, M. (2020). Midwifery students' experiences of bullying and workplace violence: A systematic review. *Midwifery, 90*, 102819–102819. https://doi.org/10.1016/j.midw.2020.102819

Cataldo, S., & Iorio, G. (Eds.). (2022). *Social love and the critical potential of people.* Routledge.

Cramer, E., & Hunter, B. (2019). Relationships between working conditions and emotional wellbeing in midwives. *Women and Birth: Journal of the Australian College of Midwives, 32*(6), 521–532. https://doi.org/10.1016/j.wombi.2018.11.010

Cronk, M. (2000). The Midwife: A professional servant? In M. Kirkham (Ed.), *The midwife-mother relationship.* Palgrave Macmillan.

Crowther, S., Cooper, C.L., Meechan, F. & Ashkanasy, N.M. (2019). The role of emotion, empathy and compassion in organisations. In S. Downe & S. Byrom (Eds.) *Squaring the circle: Normal birth research, theory and practice in a technological age* (pp. 111–119). Pinter and Martin.

Cull, J., Hunter, B., Henley, J., Fenwick, J., & Sidebotham, M. (2020). "Overwhelmed and out of my depth": Responses from early career midwives in the United Kingdom to the Work, Health and Emotional Lives of Midwives study. *Women and Birth: Journal of the Australian College of Midwives, 33*(6), e549–e557. https://doi.org/10.1016/j.wombi.2020.01.003

Di Fabio, A., & Gori, A. (2016). Assessing workplace relational civility (WRC) with a new multidimensional "Mirror" measure. *Frontiers in Psychology, 7*, 890. https://doi.org/10.3389/fpsyg.2016.00890

Di Fabio, A., & Duradoni, M. (2019). Fighting incivility in the workplace for women and for all workers: The challenge of primary prevention. *Frontiers in Psychology, 10*, 1805. https://doi.org/10.3389/fpsyg.2019.01805

Donnison. J. (1988). *Midwives and medical men. A history of the struggle for the control of childbirth* (2nd ed.). Historical Publications.

Durkheim, É. (1893). *The division of labor in society* (W. D. Halls, Trans.). Free Press.

Feeley, C. (2023). *Skilled heartfelt midwifery practice: Safe, relational care for alternative physiological births.* Springer.

Gilbert, P. (2009). *The compassionate mind.* Constable and Robinson Ltd.

Gillen, P.A., Sinclair, M., & Kernohan, W.G. (2008). The nature and manifestations of bullying in Midwifery. https://www.researchgate.net/publication/265454161_The_nature_and_manifestations_of_bullying_in_midwifery

Greenstock, K. (2023). *Flourish: A practical and emotional guidebook to thriving in midwifery*. Pinter and Martin.

Hall, J. (2013). Developing a culture of compassionate care – The midwife's voice? *Midwifery, 29*(4), 269–271. https://doi.org/10.1016/j.midw.2013.01.009

Harvie, K., Sidebotham, M., & Fenwick, J. (2019). Australian midwives' intentions to leave the profession and the reasons why. *Women and Birth: Journal of the Australian College of Midwives, 32*(6), e584–e593. https://doi.org/10.1016/j.wombi.2019.01.001

Hughes, D. (2023). Saynotobullyinginmidwifery Report. *Midwifery matters, 176*, 30.

Hunter, B., Fenwick, J., Sidebotham, M., & Henley, J. (2019). Midwives in the United Kingdom: Levels of burnout, depression, anxiety and stress and associated predictors. *Midwifery, 79*, 102526. https://doi.org/10.1016/j.midw.2019.08.008

Illouz, E. (2012). *Why love hurts: A sociological explanation*. Polity Press.

Illouz, E. (2018). *The end of love: A sociology of negative relations*. Oxford University Press.

Kirkup, B. (2015). *The report of the Morecambe Bay investigation*. https://assets.publishing.service.gov.uk/media/5a7f3d7240f0b62305b85efb/47487_MBI_Accessible_v0.1.pdf

Kirkup, B. (2022). *Reading the signals. Maternity and neonatal services in East Kent— The report of the independent investigation*. Department of Health and Social Care. https://www.gov.uk/government/publications/maternity-and-neonatal-services-in-east-kent-reading-the-signals-report

Krausé, S. S., Minnie, C. S., & Coetzee, S. K. (2020). The characteristics of compassionate care during childbirth according to midwives: A qualitative descriptive inquiry. *BMC Pregnancy and Childbirth, 20*(1), 304–304. https://doi.org/10.1186/s12884-020-03001-y

Leap, N. & Hunter, B. (2014). *The midwife's tale: an oral history from handywoman to professional midwife*. New edition. Pen & Sword Books Ltd.

Lephard, E. (2024). No more 'Us' and 'Them'. *The Practising Midwife, 27*(5), 29–31. https://doi.org/10.55975/CZMU3005

Luhmann, N. (1986). *Love as passion: The codification of intimacy* (J. Gaines & D. L. Jones, Trans.). Polity Press.

Mayra, K., Catling, C., Musa, H., Hunter, B., & Baird, K. (2023). Compassion for midwives: The missing element in workplace culture for midwives globally. *PLOS Global Public Health, 3*(7), e0002034. https://doi.org/10.1371/journal.pgph.0002034

Menage, D., Bailey, E., Lees, S., & Coad, J. (2020). Women's lived experience of compassionate midwifery: Human and professional. *Midwifery, 85*, 102662. https://doi.org/10.1016/j.midw.2020.102662

Mohammad, K. I., Al-Reda, A. N., Aldalaykeh, M., Hayajneh, W., Alafi, K. K., Creedy, D. K., & Gamble, J. (2020). Personal, professional and workplace factors associated with burnout in Jordanian midwives: A national study. *Midwifery, 89*, 102786–102786. https://doi.org/10.1016/j.midw.2020.102786

Moncrieff, G., Cheyne, H., Downe, S., & Hunter, B. (2023). Factors that influence midwives' leaving intentions: A moral imperative to intervene. *Midwifery, 125*, 103793. https://doi.org/10.1016/j.midw.2023.103793

Montagna, N. (2023). For a new sociology of social love. *The American Sociologist, 54*, 338–348. https://doi.org/10.1007/s12108-023-09572-5

NHS Leadership Academy. (2022). *Leadership listens – Introduction to the compassionate leadership miniseries*. https://learninghub.leadershipacademy.nhs.uk/leadership/leadership-listens-intro/

Nove, A., ten Hoope-Bender, P., Boyce, M., Bar-Zeev, S., de Bernis, L., Lal, G., Matthews, Z., Mekuria, M., & Homer, C. S. E. (2021). The state of the world's midwifery 2021 report: findings to drive global policy and practice. *Human Resources for Health, 19*(1), 1–146. https://doi.org/10.1186/s12960-021-00694-w

Ockenden, D. (2022). *Final report of the Ockenden review. Findings, conclusions and essential actions from the independent review of maternity services at the Shrewsbury and Telford Hospital NHS Trust*. Department of Health and Social Care. https://www.gov.uk/government/publications/final-report-of-the-ockenden-review

Patterson, J., Hollins Martin, C. J., & Karatzias, T. (2019). Disempowered midwives and traumatised women: Exploring the parallel processes of care provider interaction that contribute to women developing post traumatic stress disorder (PTSD) post childbirth. *Midwifery, 76*, 21–35. https://doi.org/10.1016/j.midw.2019.05.010

Progress Theatre. (n.d.). *Progress Theatre: supporting the work of midwives*. https://progresstheatre.wordpress.com/about/

Royal College of Midwives. (2023). *England state of maternity services 2023*. https://www.rcm.org.uk/media/6915/england-soms-2023.pdf

Sheen, K., Spiby, H., & Slade, P. (2015). Exposure to traumatic perinatal experiences and posttraumatic stress symptoms in midwives: Prevalence and association with burnout. *International Journal of Nursing Studies, 52*(2), 578–587. https://doi.org/10.1016/j.ijnurstu.2014.11.006

Smith, J. (2021). *Nurturing maternity staff: How to tackle trauma, stress and burnout to create a positive working culture in the NHS*. Pinter and Martin.

Sorokin, P. A. (1954). *The ways and power of love: Types, factors, and techniques of moral transformation*. Beacon Press.

Tam [@c3convertase]. (2024). 'I've also been bullied by midwives when I was a medical student'X 19.02.24 https://twitter.com/c3convertase/status/1759366694450164003

Teijlingen, E. (2018). *Midwives and mothers: The medicalization of childbirth on a Guatemalan plantation by Sheila Cosminsky*. Austin: University of Texas Press, 2016. 318 pp. *American Anthropologist, 120*(2), 369–369.

Uvnäs-Moberg, K. (2015). How kindness, warmth, empathy and support promote the progress of labour: A physiological perspective. In S. Byrom & S. Downe (Eds.). *The roar behind the silence: Why kindness, warmth, compassion and respect matter in maternity care* (pp. 86–93). Pinter and Martin.

Weber, M. (1922). *Economy and society: An outline of interpretive sociology* (G. Roth & C. Wittich, Eds.). University of California Press, 1978.

West, M. (2021). *Compassionate Leadership: Sustaining Wisdom, Humanity and Presence Health and Social Care*. The Swirling Leaf Press.

Winter, G. F. (2023). Bullying in the workplace. *British Journal of Midwifery, 31*(10), 597–598. https://www.britishjournalofmidwifery.com/content/comment/bullying-in-the-workplace/

Youngson, R. (2012). *Time to care. How to love your patients and your job*. Rebelheart Publishers.

Youngson, R. (2014). *The ACT with compassion coaching model*. https://www.youtube.com/watch?v=pwQ6czxFIFw

Youngson, R. (2015). We can learn to be caring. In S. Byrom & S. Downe (Eds.). *The roar behind the silence: Why kindness, warmth, compassion and respect matter in maternity care*. (pp. 67–75). Pinter and Martin.

11

LOVE IN MIDWIFERY LEADERSHIP

Michelle Waterfall

Introduction

If you complete a Google search on types of leadership, you will be over-whelmed with results. You will find words such as autocratic, democratic, transactional, transformational, laissez-faire, strategic, coaching, situational, bureaucratic; all types and styles of leadership that have been researched and written about for decades. But what you will not see in that search is love. Love is very rarely discussed or recognised as contributing to or influencing leader-ship styles. There is very little literature discussing the relationship between love and leadership. However, throughout this chapter, you will read thoughts and experiences that demonstrate that even without a huge amount of research and literature, loving leaders exist and loving leadership is being experienced by midwives in different parts of England.

Leadership

When we talk about leadership, what do we mean? Throughout the vast amount of literature surrounding leadership, there are numerous definitions of leadership, which vary greatly. From "The office or position of a leader" (Merriam-Webster, 2024), to the definition provided by Claudio Feser (co-author of Leadership at Scale) during a podcast in 2019:

> Leadership is a set of behaviours that leaders exercise to influence organisa-tional members to achieve a higher alignment on the direction that the

DOI: 10.4324/9781032645780-15

organisation is taking, to achieve a better execution of the strategy, and for the organisation to continuously renew itself.

(London, 2019)

However, if you bring together all the different elements from the numerous definitions available, leadership is really the art of guiding and inspiring people towards a shared vision or goal. It encompasses a complex set of skills, behaviours, and qualities that empower others to achieve their best potential while navigating challenges. True leadership is not about authority; it is about influence, motivation, and fostering a collaborative environment (Bass & Stogdill, 1990).

What makes a good leader?

A good leader listens attentively, communicates clearly, and empathises with their team's needs. They set a compelling vision, outlining the path forward, and encourage others to contribute their unique perspectives. A good leader demonstrates integrity by staying true to their values and making ethical decisions, even in challenging situations. Adaptability and resilience are essential traits of a leader, as they must navigate uncertainty and change, adjusting strategies as needed. What is more, a good leader fosters a culture of trust, respect, and inclusivity, valuing diversity and encouraging innovation. However, leadership is not confined to a specific role or title; it can emerge from any individual willing to take responsibility, inspire others, and drive positive change. Ultimately, an effective leader is measured by the growth, development, and success of those they lead, leaving a lasting impact on the people and organisations they work within (London, 2019; Mackey et al., 2020; Sinek, 2017). This emphasis on the growth and development of those they lead has benefits for the organisation, team, and the individual as shown in Bethan and Lisa's words.

> During my career I have been lucky enough to work within organisations that encourage compassionate and loving leadership and celebrate their staff's work and success. One of my experiences of this was being nominated by a senior leader within my division for a Trust award for outstanding contribution to care. She had taken the time to reflect upon my work and achievements and share her thanks by nominating me for my "expertise, vision, and dedication to improving services." Receiving a nomination felt fantastic! My work was visible, appreciated and recognised. I felt not only encouraged and valued, but also celebrated. Bethan, Midwife – Midlands, England.
>
> When I was a band 6 midwife working on the ward as the designated shift leader, the ward manager came to me and asked me if I had ever considered

management. She stated she had seen me organise the ward and thought I had the skills to be a manager. I had never thought about that path of career progression before and was daunted by the challenge. The ward manager put me forward for opportunities to help my development and coached me when I had doubts. 5 years later I am the Head of Midwifery! Without the ward manager tapping me on the shoulder and believing in me, I do not know if this is the path I would have taken. I felt loved because I felt seen. Someone other than myself saw my potential and encouraged my development. Lisa, Midwife – Northwest England.

Leadership in midwifery

Over the last decade leadership in midwifery has been a focus of the International Confederation of Midwives (ICM). Strengthening midwifery leadership has been a key recommendation in all three of the ICMs "State of the World's Midwifery" (SoWMy) reports. In their most recent SoWMy report (ICM, 2021), investment in midwifery leadership is acknowledged to play a key role in improving the quality and safety of sexual, reproductive, maternal, newborn, and adolescent healthcare by midwives (ICM, 2024). The ICM highlights the essential role that midwifery leadership plays in enabling midwives to work to their full potential.

The ICM recognises and prioritises midwifery leadership, ensuring it is a core element of the strategic priorities, and guarantees that the priority is recognised globally (ICM, 2024). Although having midwifery leaders in positions of authority is relatively common in European countries, the ICM highlighted that over 9% of countries have no midwives in positions of leadership in national Ministry of Health, subnational health ministry offices, regulatory authority, or health facilities. The concern is that when midwives do not hold leadership positions at health authority level, there is a significant gap in the ability of these levels of authority to provide support, oversight or mentoring to midwives and they lack the ability to make good decisions on issues that affect midwives and the care of pregnant women and their families (ICM, 2021).

Within England, we have seen a recurrent theme of ineffective leadership in maternity services being highlighted in independent inquiries into maternity services throughout the last decade (Kirkup, 2015, 2022; Ockenden, 2020, 2022). These reports also demonstrate that effective leadership is critical to establishing positive organisational culture and improving outcomes for women, and their families. This reflects the findings previously identified by the Healthcare Commission in their review of England's maternity services, highlighting the connection between not just poor clinical outcomes but also between poor workforce morale and ineffective leaderships (Alderdice et al., 2017).

In the United Kingdom, the Royal College of Midwives (RCM) reflected the ICM's recommendations when publishing Strengthening Midwifery Leadership: a manifesto to better maternity care (RCM, 2019), highlighting the vital role strong midwifery leadership has in improving maternity care. The manifesto called for steps to strengthen midwifery leadership throughout the UK National Health Service (NHS) including, having Directors of Midwifery in every trust and health board, increasing the number of consultant midwives, and strengthening and supporting midwifery education (RCM, 2019).

However, even with all the independent reports, the strategic priorities of the ICM and the RCM manifesto focusing on the importance of midwifery leadership, we are still not getting it quite right. Leadership literature talks about the qualities of a good leader being adaptive, innovative, creative, and responsive; having resilience, empathy, emotional intelligence, and the ability to foster collaboration and create vision (Ashmore et al., 2022; Knight, 2023; Warwick, 2015). But this poses the question…Where is the love?

Where is the love?

Midwifery is a caring profession. As midwives we love our profession, we love having the ability to connect with women at such a crucial and vulnerable time in their lives and having a positive impact on their pregnancy and birth journeys (Bloxsome et al., 2020). We display and feel love as midwives, so why are we not saying, "Midwifery leaders need to lead with love?".

Chapters 1 and 2 of this book show us that love is the foundation of all human existence; it shapes how we think and behave and is potentially one of our biggest motivations in life. Feeling emotions such as pride, anger, envy, and anxiety are accepted in the work environment, but love is not. Clayton (2023) investigated the reasons that love is avoided when it comes to leadership. She highlights that we consider discussing love in a work environment to be taboo, potentially making people uncomfortable. There were also concerns raised that it is seen as too intimate or even a sign of weakness. Yet in Chapter 1 of this book, we have learnt that love is connected to our human physiology and is a fundamental human function and need. Therefore, it follows that it is essential in the work environment too. Taking all of that into consideration, it makes sense that to be successful leaders we should lead with love.

Although love in leadership is not a topic that has been widely researched yet, there have been some studies and literature that consider the benefits of leading with love. They identified that leading with love naturally motivates our teams to perform at their best; it improves health and wellbeing; fosters trust and a deeper sense of emotional safety; creates cooperation, sense of togetherness and connection with others; and inspires performance, engagement, and creativity (Mielke, 2019).

How do you lead with love?

In an effort to understand more about loving leadership and how it is demonstrated, the work of Arden (2022) is valuable. Arden (2022) suggests that love is one of our biggest motivators that forms how we act and think, and her research explores why love is needed at the heart of leadership to create genuinely sustainable change. The following is developed from Arden's seven suggested ways a leader can put love at the centre of their leadership.

---

1   Start with ourselves: Build self-awareness.
2   Be open to learning: Listen, show vulnerability, be aware of weaknesses and share our mistakes – this is true not just personally as a leader, but also within our maternity services. The investigations into maternity services mentioned above have highlighted that some maternity services have not been open to learning and the negative impact this has had on the women and families that were cared for.
3   Nurture qualities of love:
    • Inclusive mindset.
    • Empathy.
    • Compassion.
    • Acceptance.
    • Understanding.
    • Curiosity.
4   Be authentic.
5   Create cultures of care: Safety and trust are created when team members can bring their whole selves to work, where they have a sense of belonging, empowered to speak up, which is key to creating psychological safety and in turn improving clinical outcomes for women and babies.
6   Stay centred in the whole system: Midwifery is an integral part of maternity and neonatal care. However, no part of maternity services can function alone, we are a system, and a loving leader recognises, engages, and empowers all parts of that system.

Jo's words below reveal the difference a loving leader can make.

Throughout my career, the relationship between love and the close intimacy of connection established and built between women, families and their midwife, has been an anchoring driver and source of great job satisfaction and pride. However, it has not been until much later in my career that I can reflect and make very similar parallels between values driven leadership approaches and behaviours that are synonymous with the founding principles of being a midwife. The ability to create trusting and empowering connections and to listen, show empathy, motivate and support are of course the same skills applied to both service users and staff alike. Core values, which include love in leadership, remain in my eyes the most powerful tool we have to create a positive and compassionate workforce.

Throughout my midwifery journey I have been privileged to feel many examples of love in leadership. The most pivotal being from my mentor and coach. From early into my career, she has always seen my potential, a person who has been willing to spend time to grow my career and have honest conversations to enable me to show up as the best version of me. She was the one that taught me how to value contributions of others openly, to recognise the importance of a compliment when best practice was demonstrated and showed me that acknowledging what other people do is the best and most authentic way to create new leaders. It mattered to me then, and it still does now, that she is proud of my achievements and of the leader I have become because she respected and cared for me as a new midwife, a midwife manager, and a midwife with potential to be a leader of the future. Jo, Midwife – Northwest England

In Chapter 2 of this book, Clare Wardhaugh writes about love having many different qualities. She uses the image of a diamond with light being reflected from many different facets, one of the facets of love being compassion. Compassion (which is discussed in more detail in Chapter 1) is an established concept in healthcare, but it is only in recent years that *compassionate leadership* has been gaining recognition. In particular, in the UK *The King's Fund* has played a pivotal role in shaping the concept of compassionate leadership within the NHS (Bailey & West, 2022; West, 2021). Compassionate leadership has grown out of a deep understanding of the complexities of healthcare environments and the importance of fostering a culture of empathy and support among healthcare professionals. In Chapter 10, the principles of compassionate leadership (attending, understanding, empathising, and helping) are discussed in the context of relationships with colleagues in maternity care settings. Importantly, West sees compassion as a manifestation of love (2021, p. 1). This is significant because it indicates that West thinks compassionate leadership *is* loving leadership (or at least a part of it), despite the reluctance to acknowledge the love found in healthcare settings. But to find examples of leadership that unashamedly profess love, it may be useful to look at other sectors.

When looking for references to love in leadership, the United States Army is not perhaps a natural place to look. However, USA army Colonel Joe Ricciardi, a decorated veteran, with three Bronze Stars and three Meritorious Service Medals from three combat tours in Afghanistan and Iraq, credits his success in leadership to love. His philosophy revolves around a profound understanding that love is not just a soft attribute but a powerful tool in leading high-performing teams and nurturing individual growth. At the core of Ricciardi's leadership style is an inherent belief in the potential of each team member. He sees beyond titles and roles, recognising the value and unique strengths that every individual member of his team brings to the table. His leadership is characterised by unwavering respect, genuine care, and a commitment to understanding the personal aspirations of his team members (Ricciardi, 2014, 2017). What is heartening is that aspects of this approach to leadership can be found in some midwifery leaders, as Tendai's words show below.

> Every day when we go to work, we wake up and work towards delivering the best care we can for our women, birthing people, families, and staff. When one has a leader who takes time to notice your passion and love for the job and they ensure that they take every opportunity to share, that means a lot. I have had the opportunity to work closely and have had ad hoc mentoring sessions due to the love of a leader to bring out my full potential. The love from a midwifery leader has been shown by respecting who I am and acknowledging the diversity I bring to the table. This love has been shown in various ways by being included in meeting agendas or discussions when no-one else thought you were needed. So, to all the midwifery leaders that stop and look around to see that individual that no one else notices, thank you. Tendai, Midwife – East of England.

Rather than relying solely on authority, Ricciardi (2017) consciously works to create an environment of trust and open communication. He achieves this through actively listening to diverse viewpoints, encouraging collaboration and creativity within his team. This instills a sense of belonging and psychological safety. The NHS England maternity services independent reports mentioned earlier (Kirkup, 2015, 2022; Ockenden 2020, 2022) found that psychological safety was not being achieved in these maternity services and that there was a negative impact on the care provided. The failures highlighted throughout the Kirkup report were born from weaknesses in culture, such as lack of teamwork, compassion, learning, and listening (Kirkup, 2022; NHS England, 2023). However, Ricciardi (2014, 2017) empowers his troops to voice their opinions without fear of judgement, creating a positive culture. It is evident from the number of publications highlighting culture in the NHS (Hancock, 2018; NHS England, 2018; NHS Improvement, 2018; NHS Resolution, 2023; The King's Fund, 2014) that in maternity services there has been a significant focus on recognising poor culture, and how to challenge it within the organisation. As a result, toolkits and guidance have been developed and even media campaigns to help raise awareness, but all the evidence demonstrates that "leadership, particularly compassionate and inclusive leadership, is the key to enabling culture changes" (NHS Improvement, 2017, p. 1, 2018).

Loving leadership can spread and grow. Anj's words below are an example of how loving leaders in midwifery inspire others to be loving leaders.

> I am a firm believer in doing everything with love and gratitude in my heart. My Grandma always said, "Be gentle, the world will make them hard," which is so true. Especially over the last five years in the world of midwifery, a global pandemic, a staffing crisis, a revolution of building resilience; a term that equates to building armour against poor behaviours, rather than spreading love, kindness, and compassion in a profession that should embody just that! In the midst of the brutal reality of the NHS I have been fortunate enough to feel love in leadership, venturing into the realms of retention, focussing on nurturing and growing the workforce, I was mentored by a senior leader who still believes in kindness, my manager, the deputy head of midwifery, no matter how pressured, always made time for a catch up and a cuppa, a chance to fill my cup, to build a solid and supportive relationship. Building a culture of psychological safety and spreading kindness, my self-worth and confidence grew, inspiring me to become a leader. A leader that leads with love, I see and feel the importance of developing bonds, of switching on connections and making sure that when I look around, I see shiny eyes looking back at me, the same ones that are born out of love. Anj, Midwife – Northwest England.

Ricciardi's (2014, 2017) research into the relationship between love and leadership, identified three factors essential to leading with love: passion, commitment, and intimacy.

Intimacy stands out as a word that is not associated with leadership in literature or in organisations. Yet, Ricciardi (2014, 2017) demonstrated that intimacy is the component with the highest value when leading with love. He believes building intimacy with your team is all about dedicating your time to understand all the members of your team on a personal level and getting to the heart of what is important to them. The key to achieving this is through authentic conversations, being genuinely curious about your team, caring about their responses and being truly invested in their wellbeing. Riccardi admits that demonstrating intimacy can be difficult and requires a leader with insight, emotional intelligence, and someone willing to invest the time with their team. In midwifery, there are many examples of leaders who know this and demonstrate it in their role, as Claire testifies below.

> When undergoing personal medical tests, I was met with such love from my manager. I had not yet told my family, but I felt that I could tell her. That is what midwifery does to you, a feeling of trust like no other. I did not require any special work requirements, or any adjustments yet, but I felt she deserved to know. I was met with such empathy and compassion, she even offered to

cover my clinical shifts! She sat and gave me her time, reflected on her own personal experiences and listened to my anxieties. I am extremely grateful to leaders like this. They are the reason I continue to practise with love and can impart this love to my patients. Claire, Midwife – West Midlands, England.

The two other components of Ricciardi's (2014, 2017) research: passion and commitment, are also fundamental but are dependent on how successfully intimacy is achieved. Passion relates to supporting team members to identify their individual and collective purpose and passion. While commitment is about commitment to the team as their leader. He proposes the question, what do you give to your team? He believes that there is a fundamental need to go above and beyond for your team (Reilly, 2021; Ricciardi, 2014, 2017).

In going above and beyond for your team, it is important to remember that a leader must also be conscious of the importance of balancing this with self-care, as discussed in Chapter 9. Leadership can be demanding and stressful, which can impact on behaviours. There are two significant ways self-care enhances a leader's ability. The first is by improving their leadership performance, maintaining the ability to show passion, commitment, and love for the whole team, and the second is through role-modelling the effects of self-care (Klug et al., 2022).

When considering how to lead with love, there is one commonality throughout all of the literature and research available: a leader's ability to lead with love being directly linked to their self-awareness and emotional intelligence. This was recognised throughout Ricciardi's research, and he is not alone in the concept. Brene Brown (2018) highlights there is significant need for leaders who are self-aware enough to lead from a place of love and she believes the key to love is allowing yourself to be vulnerable. She defines vulnerability as, "the emotion that we experience during times of uncertainty, risk, and emotional exposure" (Brown, 2018, p. 19). This is a concept that many individuals may feel does not comfortably relate to leadership. However, Brown discusses the pitfalls in not acknowledging vulnerability or pretending it does not exist, leading to fear being the main drive for thoughts and behaviour.

The emotion at the opposite end of the psychological spectrum to love is fear. Not just in the work environment but throughout society we see examples of how fear feeds and breeds fear. A leader who leads from a place of fear assumes their negative, pessimistic position is shared by others and is mirrored in their leadership style. They employ punishment, reacting rather than responding, their communication style is blunt, they will confront before understanding the facts, and will have a negative opinion they are willing to share about colleagues. If your mindset, narrative, and actions as a leader are fear-based, you become a source of fear for your team. Fear amongst leaders creates a blueprint for their team and is the central emotion for poor behaviour and cultural problems (Brown, 2020; Cook, 2020). Also, we know from the significant challenges in maternity care that poor behaviours and culture impact on a team's ability to provide high-quality, safe maternity care (Kirkup, 2015, 2022; Ockenden, 2020, 2022). The Ockenden report highlights the breakdown in communication when staff do not feel psychologically safe to escalate their concerns, especially in a culture where bullying is experienced from the top down and how this affects the care women receive (Ockenden, 2020, 2022).

A position of leadership can sometimes create a sense of loneliness (Lam et al., 2024). A leader may feel alone in the decision-making process, knowing there are potential far-reaching consequences and that they have no one to seek guidance and support from (Vidal Castelli, 2023). The sense of loneliness can also be compounded by a feeling of social isolation. As a leader moves into more senior management roles they are no longer viewed as *one of the team* and may be not included in informal team social events. Unsurprisingly, this can be hurtful and lead to loneliness and isolation. This is likely to have a negative effect on a leader, impacting their commitment, communication, and decision-making (Dierickx, 2020). It also contributes to a *us* and *them* culture with disconnect and separation between the leader and the team fostering distrust and cynicism, rather than respect and kindness (see Chapter 13 for more on the damaging effects of *us* and *them*). To actively combat this type of loneliness, a leader needs emotional intelligence and the ability to consciously put coping strategies in place. Spelman (2024) advises creating a network of leaders to cultivate connections within their professional community; increasing peer learning: working with a mentor, building cohesion within the team through fun, engaging in social activities, maintaining a personal friendship circle, and ensuring a healthy work–life balance is maintained.

Everybody needs to feel that they belong and that they are cared about. Leaders are no exception. They need love too.

Why is leading with love important in midwifery?

The wellbeing of the midwifery workforce has been a concern raised for many years. The challenge has been highlighted through a growing body of evidence demonstrating increased levels of emotional distress contributing to low morale, burnout, and midwifery attrition (RCM, 2016a; Leversidge, 2016; RCM, 2016b; Sheen et al., 2015; Yoshida & Sandall, 2013). To compound these concerns, there have been significant workforce challenges, which have impacted further on the health and wellbeing of midwives. In England, we are currently experiencing higher rates of absence from work categorised as mental health concerns, than ever before. However, research shows that employees who felt their working environment was one of a loving culture reported greater satisfaction in their roles and better teamwork. There were lower rates of sickness and absence. People who worked in a loving culture also felt able to express their affection, tenderness, caring, and compassion for their colleagues, were also more satisfied and committed to the organisation, and felt a greater sense of accountability for their performance (Barsade & O'Neil, 2014). In an environment like the NHS, with significant financial pressures and limited resources, leading with love can make a difference, creating a motivated, well supported, and caring team despite the adversity and financial restrictions faced (Lee & Mahaniah, 2021).

It is not just the workforce that is affected by loving leadership. Loving leadership also has a positive impact on the outcome of the care we provide for women and their families. Research suggests there are links between positive relational leadership, such as love, and an increase in patient satisfaction as well as reduced levels of patient mortality, medication errors, hospital-acquired infections, and length of stay (Wong et al., 2013). Although the research was conducted in nursing environments, it is possible to draw the direct comparison to midwifery care. Savannah's words below are testimony to the positive impact that loving midwifery leadership can have.

> To experience love from a midwifery leader is a feeling of belonging. It is knowing you are valued, appreciated and safe to express your ideas and opinions. Love from a midwifery leader gave me the confidence to question, to develop, to make change; whilst knowing she would support me with kindness along my journey. Savannah, Midwife – Northwest England.

When love is shown in this way, it spreads and eventually its impact is evident in the whole team providing midwifery care. Little by little it will spread and change the whole culture. This loving environment will filter through to improve the experience of women and families in our care (Barsade & O'Neil, 2014).

Chapter takeaways

Drawing on the work of Brown (2018), Mielke (2019), and Ricciardi (2014, 2017), the following provide a summary of an approach to leading with love in midwifery.

LEADING WITH LOVE IS A MINDSET AND CHOICE

Leading with love is an act and needs action to demonstrate it.
  To lead with love, you need to -

- **Understand and care** about the things that empower, motivate and are significant to your team.

- **Create deeper connection** with your team, through team building, one-to-one sessions, social activities or any activity that creates quality time together.
- **Be vulnerable**, show weaknesses and share mistakes, this will allow your team to be vulnerable too.
- **Recognise achievements** of individuals within your team, validate their unique qualities, abilities, or successes in a personal way, for example, handwritten cards of gratitude.
- **Create time** for each individual team member through dedicated, uninterrupted one-to-one time. Whether this is through a catch-up over a coffee or a more formal one-to-one setting; this needs empathetic listening, open body language, and communication. It is important to turn your computer off, put your phone away and give 100% of yourself.

References

Alderdice, F., Bannon, E.M., & McNeills, J. (2017). A review of midwifery leadership. *British Journal of Midwifery*, 25(10), 655–661. https://doi.org/10.12968/bjom.2017.25.10.655

Arden, Z. (2022). *Why we need to put love at the heart of our leadership.* https://zoearden.com/insights/why-we-need-to-put-love-at-the-heart-of-our-leadership

Ashmore, A. A., Kanga, K., Kaur-Desai, T., Thorman, K., & Archer, N. (2022). Building leadership capabilities in maternity. *BMJ Leader*, 6(1), 10–14. https://doi.org/10.1136/leader-2021-000449

Bailey, S., & West, M. (2022). *What is compassionate leadership?* The King's Fund. https://www.kingsfund.org.uk/insight-and-analysis/long-reads/what-is-compassionate-leadership

Barsade, S., & O'Neil, O. A. (2014). *Employees who feel love perform better.* Harvard Business Review https://hbr.org/2014/01/employees-who-feel-love-perform-better

Bass, B. M., & Stogdill, R. M. (1990). *Bass and Stogdill's handbook of leadership* (3rd ed.). Free Press.

Bloxsome, D., Bayes, S., & Ireson, D. (2020). "I love being a midwife; it's who I am": A Glaserian grounded theory study of why midwives stay in midwifery. *Journal of Clinical Nursing*, 29(1–2), 208–220. https://doi.org/10.1111/jocn.15078

Brown, B. (2018). *Dare to lead.* Penguin Random House UK.

Brown, B. (2020). *The gift of imperfection: Let go of who you think you're supposed to be and embrace who you are.* (2nd ed.). Penguin Random House UK.

Clayton, H. (2023). *Leading from love.* https://helenaclayton.co.uk/wp-content/uploads/2019/11/Leading-with-Love-White-Paper-v2.pdf

Cook, J. (2020). *Why you should lead with love and not fear.* Thrive Global. https://www.forbes.com/sites/jodiecook/2020/05/11/love-or-fear/

Dierickx, C. (2020). *Why loneliness is a problem for leaders and what to do about it.* https://www.forbes.com/sites/constancedierickx/2020/06/23/why-loneliness-is-a-problem-for-leaders-and-what-to-do-about-it/

Hancock, M. (2018). *Good NHS leadership starts with culture change.* Department of Health and Social Care. https://www.gov.uk/government/speeches/good-nhs-leadership-starts-with-culture-change

International Confederation of Midwives. (2021). *The state of the world's midwifery.* International Confederation of Midwives. https://www.unfpa.org/sites/default/files/pub-pdf/21-038-UNFPA-SoWMy2021-Report-ENv4302.pdf

International Confederation of Midwives. (2024). *A guide for midwifery leadership.* International Confederation of Midwives. https://internationalmidwives.org/resources/guide-for-midwifery-leadership/

Kirkup, B. (2015). *Morecambe bay investigation: Report.* Morecambe Bay Investigation. https://www.gov.uk/government/publications/morecambe-bay-investigation-report

Kirkup, B. (2022). *Maternity and neonatal services in East Kent: 'Reading the signals' report.* Department of Health and Social care. https://www.gov.uk/government/publications/maternity-and-neonatal-services-in-east-kent-reading-the-signals-report

Klug, K., Felfe, J., & Krick, A. (2022). Does self-care make you a better leader? A multi-source study linking leader self-care to health-oriented leadership, employee self-care, and health. *International Journal of Environmental Research and Public Health, 19*(11), 6733. https://doi.org/10.3390/ijerph19116733

Knight, R. (2023). *8 essential qualities of a successful leader.* Harvard Business Review. https://hbr.org/2023/12/8-essential-qualities-of-successful-leaders

Lam, H., Giessner, S. R., Shemla, M., Werner, M. D. (2024). Leader and leadership loneliness: A review-based critique and path to future research. *The Leadership Quarterly, 35*(3), 101780. https://doi.org/10.1016/j.leaqua.2024.101780

Lee, P. T., & Mahaniah, K. J. (2021). Leading with love: Five practical tips. *Journal of General Internal Medicine, 36*(11), 3530–3531. https://doi.org/10.1007/s11606-021-06768-8

Leversidge, A. (2016). Why midwives leave – Revisited. *Midwives, 19*(Winter),19.

London, S. (Host). (2019, Feb 28). What is leadership: Moving beyond the C-Suite. [Audio Podcast episode]. *McKinskey Podcast.* Mckinskey & Company. https://www.mckinsey.com/featured-insights/leadership/what-is-leadership

Mackey, J., McIntosh, S., & Phillips, C. (2020). *Conscious leadership: Elevating humanity through business.* Penguin.

Merriam-Webster. (2024). https://www.google.com/search?q=Leadership+Definition+%26+Meaning+-+Merriam-Webster&oq=Leadership+Definition+%26+Meaning+-+Merriam-Webster&gs_lcrp=EgZjaHJvbWUyBggAEEUYOdIBBzgzN2owajSoAgCwAgE&sourceid=chrome&ie=UTF-8

Mielke, A. (2019). *5 reasons why innovative leaders lead with love.* Linkedin. https://www.linkedin.com/pulse/5-reasons-why-innovative-leaders-lead-love-ashley-mielke

NHS England. (2018). A just culture guide. https://www.england.nhs.uk/patient-safety/patient-safety-culture/a-just-culture-guide/#about-our-guide

NHS England. (2023). *Three-year delivery plan for maternity and neonatal services.* https://www.england.nhs.uk/wp-content/uploads/2023/03/B1915-three-year-delivery-plan-for-maternity-and-neonatal-services-march-2023.pdf

NHS Improvement. (2017). *Why is culture important?* https://www.england.nhs.uk/wp-content/uploads/2021/06/01-NHS101-02-Improvement-Mini-Guide-Why-100417-I.pdf

NHS Improvement. (2018, March 15). A just culture guide. [Video]. YouTube. https://www.youtube.com/watch?v=zje765OEggs

NHS Resolution. (2023). *Being fair 2. Promoting a person-centred workplace that is compassionate, safe and fair.* https://resolution.nhs.uk/resources/being-fair-2/

Ockenden, D. (2020). *Emerging findings and recommendations from the independent review of maternity services at the Shrewsbury and Telford Hospital NHS trust.* Department of Health and Social Care. https://www.gov.uk/government/publications/ockenden-review-of-maternity-services-at-shrewsbury-and-telford-hospital-nhs-trust

Ockenden, D. (2022). *Final report of the Ockenden review. Findings, conclusions and essential actions from the independent review of maternity services at the Shrewsbury and Telford Hospital NHS Trust.* Department of Health and Social Care. https://www.gov.uk/government/publications/final-report-of-the-ockenden-review

Reilly, C. (2021). *Leaders of love: Transforming the workplace.* Forbes.com. https://www.forbes.com/sites/colleenreilly/2021/02/10/leaders-of-love-transforming-the-workplace/

Ricciardi, J. (2014, Dec 14). *At the intersection of love and leadership.* [Video]. Youtube. https://youtu.be/nV8_0kt2VVg?feature=shared

Ricciardi, J. (2017, Aug 30). *War, love and leadership.* [Video]. Vimeo. https://vimeo.com/231719418

Royal College of Midwives. (2016a). *Why midwives leave – Revisited.* https://cdn.ps.emap.com/wp-content/uploads/sites/3/2016/10/Why-Midwives-Leave.pdf

Royal College of Midwives. (2016b). *Caring for you campaign: Survey results. RCM campaign for healthy workplaces delivering high quality care.* RCM.com. rcm-campaign-for-healthy-workplaces-delivering-high-quality-care-caring-for-you-survey-results.pdf

Royal College of Midwives. (2019). *Strengthen midwifery leadership: A manifesto for better maternity care.* RCM. https://pre.rcm.org.uk/media/3527/strengthening-midwifery-leadership-a4-12pp_7-online-3.pdf

Sheen, K., Spiby, H., & Slade, P. (2015). Exposure to traumatic perinatal experiences and posttraumatic stress symptoms in midwives: Prevalence and association with burnout. *International Journal of Nursing Studies, 52*(2), 578–587. https://doi.org/10.1016/j.ijnurstu.2014.11.006

Sinek, S. (2017). *Leaders eat last.* Penguin Random House UK.

Spelman, E. (2024). *Leadership over Loneliness: How unleashing the leader within transformed my life.* Independently Published.

The King's Fund. (2014). *Improving NHS culture.* https://www.kingsfund.org.uk/insight-and-analysis/projects/improving-nhs-culture

Vidal Castelli, P. (2023). *The burden of leadership: Addressing loneliness.* https://www.forbes.com/councils/forbescoachescouncil/2023/05/03/the-burden-of-leadership-addressing-loneliness/

Warwick, C., (2015). *Leadership in maternity services: The health foundation, inspiring movement.* Health Foundation.

West, M. (2021). *Compassionate leadership: Sustaining wisdom, humanity and presence health and social care.* The Swirling Leaf Press.

Wong, C. A., Cummings, G. G., & Ducharme, L. (2013). The relationship between nursing leadership and patient outcomes: A systematic review update. *Journal of Nursing Management, 21*(5), 709–724. https://doi.org/10.1111/jonm.12116

Yoshida, Y., & Sandall, J. (2013). Occupational burnout and work factors in community and hospital midwives: A survey analysis. *Midwifery*, 29(8), 921–926. https://doi.org/10.1016/j.midw.2012.11.002

12

LOVE IN MIDWIFERY EDUCATION

Maeve O'Connell and Naomi O'Donovan

Introduction

In this chapter, I (Maeve) reflect on and discuss the role of love in midwifery education. My conversations with fellow midwifery educator (Naomi) have been pivotal in recognising how love appears and enhances our work, and Naomi's experiences are important contributions within the chapter. Although we work in different countries, systems, and cultures (I in the United Arab Emirates and Naomi in Ireland), we have both experienced loving midwifery education as a force for good.

As I began to write, my belief that love is inherent in midwifery education was challenged as I tried to reconcile my role as educator with the term *love*, which is commonly associated with intimacy or romance. However, love is much broader than this. Following several exploratory conversations, I understand that while in nursing literature discussions around love are not unusual, they remain very limited within midwifery. Yet, in the current climate of increasing fear of childbirth and birth trauma, emotional burnout, stress due to short staffing, and the isolation and suffering from the COVID-19 pandemic, a discussion on love is much needed.

This chapter explores aspects of loving midwifery education while also considering the ethical, moral, and regulatory standards around midwifery. The aim is to guide the reader in their individual reflective journey as a midwife, midwifery student, or educator, to consider the role of love in midwifery education. There are reflective questions and learning points to help critical thinking and readers can use these to write a reflection or keep a journal.

DOI: 10.4324/9781032645780-16

Chapter 1 of this book explored some of the different sorts of love and some of these resonated with my role as a midwifery educator. I open this chapter by discussing some of these in relation to my role.

Forms of love within midwifery education

Agape

Reflecting on our roles as midwifery educators, Naomi and I considered the notion of unconditional love or *agape* love, as selfless, unconditional love for all beings. I thought about how this can be expressed in midwifery education. At surface level, education encompasses teaching, learning, and assessment to ensure competent practitioners but alongside this it requires a compassionate and positive learning culture underpinned by unconditional love. However, creating this culture is complex and challenging. Nevertheless, agape is a broad charitable love for humanity where equality, ethical treatment, and respect for persons is borne. This love aligns with the UK Nursing and Midwifery Council (NMC) code on dignity and upholding human rights (NMC, 2018) and is therefore ideally suited for midwifery education.

Ludus

Naomi reminded me that my educator role connects with the playful form of love the Greeks called *Ludus*. This arises in the shared experiences of learning in the skills lab and simulations, where students giggle and may be hesitant to participate. University clinical skills suites are designed for learning midwifery skills and practising clinical competencies, where mistakes can be made and corrected, with no harm. Students practise skills amongst peers and are debriefed after emergency drills. This builds confidence and diminishes anxiety around participating in obstetric emergencies (Vermeulen et al., 2021). Naomi shared that she has experienced lovely moments where awkwardness was replaced with liberation and fun, and I was quizzed in return. I frequently advocate Confucius' principle that "A man who has committed a mistake and doesn't correct it is committing another mistake" (Confucius, Chinese philosopher & reformer, 551 BC–479 BC). Naomi told me that she reminds students that she once used an incorrect instrument to clamp an umbilical cord and the midwife she was working with laughingly said "Well, you'll never do that again will you?". Midwifery students articulate a need for safe spaces to learn with those who are invested in their clinical placement learning; educators in an academic setting must equally fulfil this requirement (Neiterman et al., 2022). Patiently sharing knowledge, kindly correcting, and gently encouraging students in their skills labs is an inherently loving pedagogy. Simulations and drills afford the students opportunities to reflect on a variety of interpersonal interactions, communication, and teamwork outside of the pressures of the clinical settings.

Storge

Working as a midwife exposes you to love on multiple levels: the intimate private love of partners, the love of parents for their newborn, the tentative (sometimes reluctant) love of a sibling for a new baby. We are intrinsically linked to *storge* (the Greek term for familial love) when we initiate skin to skin and support a new mother feeding or reassure a new family that they are doing well. We guide and encourage while providing clear boundaries and applying evidence-based knowledge such as advising on safe sleep or cord care.

Our reflections on agape, ludus, and storge left me feeling foolish for being reticent to see the love in our work as educators. In fact, we must apply a loving pedagogy to prepare students to work in an arena where very raw, real love exists and must be allowed to flourish.

How midwifery education has developed

Traditionally, midwifery education, like nursing, was provided through apprenticeship models in a task-oriented, regimented style. Often, midwifery followed on from nursing to develop all round competent healthcare professionals, as was the case in Ireland, where I was one of the last students to experience nursing training provided by nuns. This relied heavily on didactic pedagogies of learning where the focus was on teachers delivering lessons as opposed to student-led learning. Our education moved to the university during my time, and I recall occasions when clinical supervisors would embarrass students or reprimand them publicly in the name of high standards and expectations of care. Most of my clinical midwifery mentors would have trained in this model of education where learning happened *on the job* and a strict hierarchy of staff dominated. Today, globally, midwifery training is increasingly located in universities as a degree programme, a shift thought to improve attractiveness of the training and autonomy of the profession (Migura, 2024). This happened in the early 2000s in Ireland and the United Kingdom, more recently in Austria, Switzerland, and Canada. In Germany, the shift from vocational schools to higher institutions only occurred in 2023 (Migura, 2024). Universities employ student-centred approaches to learning that aid critical thinking, which is particularly useful in health and social care. However, in many countries, midwifery education remains outside of universities, often as a specialised branch of nursing (Sharif et al., 2021).

Contemporary education approaches assist the student to critically reflect on care given and to receive useful feedback to gain an insight into how to improve practice or behaviour. Sometimes students have a particular barrier to learning or there may be a sudden change in behaviour. There are many possible reasons why this could happen including personal issues and bullying. Educators need to consider this and provide supervision directing students to appropriate support that may be available in the university. When we lovingly and compassionately approach students facing challenges with their learning, we can identify the aspect (cognitive, psychomotor, or affective) that needs to be addressed and create an action plan. Thus, just as midwives should tailor healthcare to meet women's unique needs, mentors should adapt their teaching methods to suit the learning style of each student to support them to succeed.

REFLECTION FOR MIDWIVES, MIDWIFE EDUCATORS, CLINICAL SUPERVISORS, AND MIDWIFERY STUDENTS

- In what ways is love required in midwifery education?
- Are you experiencing or did you experience a loving education environment as a midwifery student?
- What challenges are you facing, or did you face in your midwifery education, especially when it comes to balancing your love for the field with the difficulties you've encountered?

Relationships in midwifery education

Rae Rudinski, a teacher frequently quoted for her educational philosophy said,

> Be consistent, but flexible. Love them unconditionally but hold them accountable. Give them a voice, but be their leader.
>
> *(Rudinski, n.d., as cited in Elias, 2016)*

This quote depicts the tension between students and educators, where compassion (a facet of love discussed in Chapters 1 and 2) is required, alongside accountability for actions or inaction and the need to lead students to reach their potential. In essence, the quote demonstrates the dynamic nature of love and how a balance between compassion, support, and guidance may help students thrive. In midwifery education, we advocate for our student midwives, and we also lead with love and compassion.

Midwifery student–educator relationships develop during time spent together teaching and learning. However, large midwifery cohorts, often of more than one hundred students may lessen this personal experience in what is a particularly challenging programme. For many students, challenges include being young and just finding their feet in the world as an adult, and lack of experience and confidence. Furthermore, increasing complexity and medicalisation of maternity may lead to challenges in achieving the required midwifery competencies (that focus on physiological birth). Many students also face financial, housing, and mental health problems (Carolan-Olah et al., 2014; Fenwick et al., 2016). Nevertheless, in my experience, a bond between midwifery educators and students often develops and many of my students have said "I will never forget you and the influence you had on my life." I certainly hold a special place in my heart for the midwives who educated me across theory and in clinical practice and have stayed in touch with many of them. However, positive experiences are not always the case and negative, unsupportive relationships during a student's pre-registration education can be damaging.

We witness our students developing, both personally and professionally, and it is truly incredible to see. The journey from first year to graduation is far from linear; students must face and overcome many personal and academic challenges, becoming very different people, shaped not just by their education but by the love and encouragement they receive along the way. Love and compassion, expressed through encouraging words and actions, are integral in supporting students through their journey. The specific role of the personal tutor/advisor in providing pastoral care is invaluable, offering the support and guidance needed to help students navigate difficult circumstances and achieve their goals. Through a nurturing environment, students are empowered to overcome obstacles and emerge as confident, capable midwives.

Enabling students: professional boundaries, socialisation, and identities

Midwives work in highly gendered, often hierarchical environments, with global variation in midwifery autonomy, often challenged through medicalisation (Neiterman et al., 2024). Professional boundaries are usually established through formal regulatory channels, to ensure care remains both ethical and empathetic, yet boundaries are often unclear, and remain underexplored in research (Neiterman et al., 2024). The scope of practice, outlined by curricula and practice guidelines, helps maintain a balance between compassionate care and professional responsibility. Professional socialisation concentrates on how students adopt and internalise professional identities and values, with the understanding that establishing boundaries is vital for learning and to practise their profession effectively (Neiterman et al., 2024). Professional socialisation empowers students to reshape and redefine professional boundaries, so they transition from being mere learners to becoming active agents of change within their profession, contributing to the evolution and improvement of practice standards. Boundaries are always important in relationships whether professional or personal. Professional boundaries ensure that caring relationships can be navigated safely for all parties (see a section on boundaries in Chapter 13) and supporting student midwives with setting and maintaining appropriate professional boundaries is an important part of midwifery education.

Lovingly supporting self-care

Self-care is an important concept to include in midwifery curricula, encouraging self-love, compassion, and love for others. This is discussed in more depth in Chapter 9 which discussed strategies for self-care comprehensively. However, it is included in this chapter as it is so important to embed this concept from the very start.

Midwifery education can play an important part in helping students to gain the confidence and skills they need to maintain their health and wellbeing. An understanding of how to maintain a healthy work–life balance and self-awareness strategies can be taught. Tools to deal with academic pressures, and the stress they will inevitably encounter in the clinical environment, can be developed and honed if embedded into the curriculum. For example, it is not unusual for students to report that they did not have time or opportunity for a break on a shift. Taking breaks is not only vital for wellbeing but we know that midwives often ignore their own needs, placing the needs of work as a priority and working over their contracted hours because of staffing needs.

Preparing students to maintain their right to a break involves advocacy and empowerment. Educators can advocate for students to ensure that supervisors and mentors respect and uphold these rights. They can also empower students by equipping them with the tools and confidence to advocate for themselves. This can include teaching students effective communication and assertiveness skills, not just in theory but by providing safe spaces to role-play different scenarios, practising uncomfortable conversations. By balancing advocacy with empowerment, educators can help students navigate these situations in the clinical area with confidence and integrity.

REFLECTION FOR MIDWIVES, MIDWIFE EDUCATORS, CLINICAL SUPERVISORS

- As educators, how can we prepare students to maintain their right to a break?
- How can we advocate for students and equip them with the tools to advocate for themselves?

However, there are many barriers to self-care and students need to be able to recognise these. Naomi's words below provide an example of facilitating learning around self-care and self-awareness.

When teaching health promotion, I ask the students to give examples of what they think they should do for their wellbeing. We compile lists of actions and behaviours that are good for us. Then I ask them if they do them all or which one they wish to aspire to most? Invariably the students will arrive at sleep, hygiene, improving diet or exercise, mental health, and wellbeing practices such as meditation. I try to offer the opportunity to arrive at a compassionate perspective and open their eyes to why with all their knowledge and self-efficacy they cannot improve diet/sleep/activity or give up smoking or reduce alcohol intake. It also raises awareness of the inequalities that exist among the group e.g., those with responsibilities of caring for children or family or those who have a lengthy commute. We can remember these activities when we identify and discuss the difficulties faced by different socioeconomic groups or the global majority populations. The aim in my teaching of health promotion is to activate students' self-awareness and encourage empathy towards themselves and the women they care for in addition to their own theoretical knowledge.

Naomi's words above demonstrate a loving, guided activity with students which helps them to see that knowing what to do is not enough. This supportive group activity encourages students to reflect on and discuss the practical, emotional, social, and cultural challenges regarding self-care, for themselves and others, and to reflect on them.

The nature of the learning environment

Environment has been mentioned above but here it is explored more fully. The nature of the learning environment directly impacts students' development. Knowledge, skills, and behaviours are best developed in positive learning environments (Adam et al., 2021). If we want midwifery students to learn, flourish, and thrive, a supportive clinical learning environment is not just beneficial, it is essential (Adam et al., 2021). A positive and nurturing atmosphere cultivates confidence, encourages engagement, and ultimately leads to better outcomes in both education and practice. Given the pressures that midwives face (short staffing, stressful clinical environments), midwifery educators want to seek ways to ensure midwifery students feel safe and supported when in clinical placement.

How we as people treat each other has a huge influence on the way we feel in any environment, whether that be in the classroom, lecture theatre or in the clinical setting. A systematic review by Keller et al. (2020) shows that incivility is now recognised as not just being thoughtless or unkind but as having an impact on patient safety, with examples of incivility, including rudeness, disruptive behaviours, interpersonal tensions, gossip, and treating people as if they were invisible. Situational and cultural factors associated with increased levels of incivility include heavy workloads, communication and coordination problems, patient safety issues, lack of support, and inadequate leadership (Keller et al., 2020). Interventions for addressing incivility and unprofessional behaviour include education and policy (Russell, 2014). Understanding the impact of uncivil behaviour and developing effective communication strategies is important in maintaining professionalism (Russell, 2014). Focusing on teamwork, leadership, and conflict management strategies are recommended to equip students with the relevant skills and behaviours. Exploring the reasons for incivility and ways of dealing with it are important parts of midwifery education.

REFLECTION FOR MIDWIVES, MIDWIFE EDUCATORS, CLINICAL SUPERVISORS, AND MIDWIFERY STUDENTS

- What is or has been your experience of incivility in the workplace?
- How do you think midwifery educators can prepare students to navigate and respond to incivility?
- What role does loving support from educators play in helping students thrive in these situations?

We should aspire to a loving workplace culture, where staff find meaning and purpose in their work and feel valued and psychologically safe. Yet, incivility and bullying are prevalent. A report by Barrett et al. (2023) called #saynotobullyinginmidwifery has given an insight into the types of culture of incivility which have pervaded midwifery. Midwives of diverse backgrounds and experiences contributed their stories, from student midwives and newly qualified to those with decades of experience. Midwives who contributed stories to the report felt "undervalued and not listened to"; reported "being treated like a slave"; "bullying, unkind and unprofessional behaviours in a culture of exhaustion, feeling demoralised and stressed"; "belittling and ageism"; "collusion and gaslighting"; and "racism and religious discrimination" (Barrett et al., 2023). Many of these newly qualified midwives left the profession within a year of qualification and reported a deterioration in their mental health. Psychological distress and burnout are consistently reported as prevalent in midwifery (Hunter et al., 2019; Pezaro et al., 2016). A lack of respect for midwifery specialism was revealed where highly trained professionals experienced disrespect (Barrett et al., 2023).

Students should feel loved and valued during their clinical placements to meet their fundamental human need for fulfilment. According to Maslow's Hierarchy of Needs (Maslow, 1954), after basic needs of safety, security, and physiological requirements, individuals have a deep-seated need for love, belonging, and self-esteem. When students experience genuine care and appreciation from their mentors and peers, they are more likely to feel a sense of belonging and self-worth. This supportive environment not only enhances their learning experience but also nurtures their personal and professional growth. Meeting this need for emotional support and recognition is crucial for students to thrive, as it helps them achieve higher levels of motivation, confidence, and overall satisfaction in their roles. This starts with feeling welcomed by staff who use their first names. Role modelling professional behaviours is vital because for students it is a key aspect of learning what it is to be a midwife. Recognising when someone is excelling and calling out good practice is motivational. Equally, delivering negative feedback, while difficult, can be done lovingly by being both constructive and compassionate, encouraging students rather than shaming them.

A note on giving feedback lovingly

When providing feedback, plan the conversation and make space to deliver feedback in privacy at a mutually convenient time. Students should understand what is required and if they are not meeting requirements understand why not. A specific action plan is useful to guide students to pass at the next assessment opportunity. Timely feedback is important; concerns about the student's performance should be raised with the student as soon as possible, rather than waiting for an assessment point. This ensures equity and fairness so that insight into how to improve is possible.

Learning point: A positive clinical learning environment is vital to enhance student learning and wellbeing. When students feel valued as a member of the team, learning is optimised.

REFLECTION FOR MIDWIVES, MIDWIFE EDUCATORS, CLINICAL SUPERVISORS

- How do you create a welcoming and supportive environment for midwifery students when they first enter the clinical area?
- What strategies or resources do you use to help them feel prepared and informed?
- What sort of feedback helps students to learn and be accountable to provide safe and competent care?
- How can we ensure that midwifery students experience quality supervision in clinical placements?

Reflection for Students

- What helps you feel welcomed and supported in the clinical environment?
- What are your experiences of receiving feedback?

Using creativity to reflect on the joy of midwifery

Reflective practice is an important component of midwifery pre-registration education (Sweet et al., 2019) and beyond, and the skills required to become a reflective practitioner are embedded in the UK NMC revalidation process (NMC, 2018). Critical reflection on a situation can shed light on why and how events unfolded, so that students can learn and move forward. Most student midwives are familiar with academic reflective writing, but less formal private reflection and journaling can also assist students to make sense of their experiences.

Arts-based pedagogy can allow midwifery students to develop new perspectives and then to attribute meaning to some of the profound experiences they encounter (Obara et al., 2022). Naomi incorporates art and creativity into her teaching which she finds helpful for students to build relationships, and a sense of not being alone. Now a midwifery educator, Naomi as a student reflected on a particular occasion on a clinical placement when she was supported to be truly *with woman*. Naomi wrote the following poem, as a reflective tool.

WITH WOMAN

I missed the conception – the sweet pain, the writhing, the sweat and moans, and the ecstasy.

During the bearing I have not been there either.

But I am here now. I am with you.

Woman do not fear, come with me. Together we will come to a place of joy.

I will guide you through churning waters and bring you to harbour.

To shore.

And when the moon calls me again, I will go back out to the wild to seek another soul to bring to safety.

To Bliss. Fulfilment.

In the blue scrubs and bright lights I am with you. Woman I am here with you.

In the flurry of injections, cord traction and machines that go beep, and pip and squeak.

I am with you – stars in darkness, roiling black waters.

Sweet pain, writhing sweat, moaning and glorious actualisation.

Take my hand, my heart. I am yours for as long as you need me.

So sweet woman, come to shore. To the culmination of love and hope.

Rivulets of blood and perspiration. Ruddy cheeks and eyes bright.

Days swim into night.

We are of the world and out of it.

Foreheads pressed. Whispering. Strength and gentleness meld, melt and merge.

Pushing, panting, gasping, smiling, crying, laughing, and perfect, perfect joy.

And as your needs release me I am not sure which one of us floats from the other.

Yet I will always be with you.

When reflecting back on writing the poem, Naomi said,

> I vividly remember the night I wrote about in my poem *With Woman*. It was an extremely busy night on the birthing suite. I joined a Domino midwife (a member of a small team of midwives providing continuity) in a room with a multiparous woman who was very distressed, but Mags (my preceptor) let me try to calm and reassure her. She and I connected with touch and voice and breath. It was a very profound moment and after the birth I went back to the busy corridor and through the window had a flash of boats as it was night and we were near the harbour at home in West Cork. It felt like I was on a mission, not to rescue but to bring the women to that safe place of birth. It makes me now stand back to allow the students to take my place which I lovingly surrender to them.

Reflections do not always come naturally to students and real-life clinical practice post qualification does not afford much value to this important practice. Academic style reflections certainly have a place but diminishing the focus on the *art* of midwifery causes a chasm to emerge whereby some students grapple to deal with the emotive and deeply personal work of a midwife. Using more spontaneous, creative approaches to reflection such as a narrative pedagogical approach, namely storytelling, can enhance learning and humanises the experience (Gilkison et al., 2016).

Virtues versus values

Values are ideals, goals, or beliefs that allow us to make judgements about what is right and wrong. Virtues are those values in action. A value becomes a virtue when it is demonstrated in real life. The concepts of virtues and values are deeply interconnected, with their origins rooted in the philosophy of Aristotle. Aristotle introduced the concept of *flourishing* (eudaimonia), emphasising that achieving a fulfilling and meaningful life requires the cultivation of virtues such as courage, temperance, and wisdom. These virtues are seen as essential for living a life of moral excellence and personal satisfaction. In contemporary times, many professional values, such as integrity, respect, and empathy, are influenced by Aristotle's work. Modern ethical frameworks and professional standards often reflect these principles and are integral to guiding professional conduct and personal development (Groothuizen et al., 2018). Kuipers (2022) has explored virtues in woman-centred care and has identified eighteen virtues; notably one of these is love.

Values-based recruitment has become a global priority for healthcare and has been embedded in recruitment processes following multiple reports of care deficiencies worldwide, but particularly in the UK since the landmark Mid Staffordshire report (Francis, 2013; Spilsbury et al., 2022). Consequently, the NHS has embraced a values-based approach to recruitment of midwives and nurses with the aim of emphasising the need for compassionate care (Groothuizen et al., 2018; Power & Clews, 2015). Future NHS professionals are recruited based on their alignment with NHS Constitution Values, which are: working together for patients, respect and dignity, commitment to quality, compassion, improving lives, and everyone counts.

This approach begins during the educational recruitment process, where assessing a candidate's suitability for the profession involves evaluating their commitment to the quality of care, respect, dignity, and their genuine love for improving lives. The approach has been criticised on the basis that the recruitment of the *right people* places too much emphasis on personal characteristics, rather than focussing on the systemic problems with healthcare (Groothuizen et al., 2018). However, the care failings highlighted in the Francis Report (Francis, 2013) were rooted in a culture focused more on *doing the system's business* rather than truly caring for patients with love and compassion. This observation suggests that the failings in care may not be solely due to the personal characteristics or values of healthcare professionals, but rather the pressures and demands of the healthcare system itself. A love-driven approach to recruitment and care must consider not only the personal qualities of healthcare workers but also the environment and systems in which they operate. For example, the virtue of courage is important because it takes courage to stand up to what is not right and ensure that caring for people always comes before doing the system's business.

Building loving midwifery programmes using Universal Design for Learning (UDL)

Ensuring the parity of opportunity and experience for all students, including mature students, students of different abilities and from different socioeconomic and cultural backgrounds, is a cornerstone of contemporary higher education. When all educators adopt this approach, the experience of students is optimised. Many universities now embed the UDL principles and guidance across all courses to ensure that all learners can access and take part in meaningful and valuable learning opportunities. It is based on evidence-based insights into how human brains work with the aim of engaging all students, optimising their learning (CAST, 2024). When used in midwifery education, it can be seen as a set of loving and compassionate principles that help midwifery educators meet students' needs, profoundly enhancing their learning experience. The three key principles are described below.

The first principle, the *why* **of learning**, emphasises the importance of understanding the motivation behind why students should learn. By providing multiple means of engagement, educators can foster a loving and supportive environment that inspires students to be genuinely interested and invested in their education (University College Cork [UCC], 2021). For example, using stories and personal experiences to connect theoretical knowledge with real-world practice can make learning more meaningful. However, recognising that some learners might face cultural barriers or personal fears is crucial. In the Middle East, for instance, students might feel uncomfortable with certain anatomical images due to cultural sensitivities. Addressing these concerns with empathy and patience, explaining the importance of understanding anatomy for effective midwifery care, helps students overcome these barriers, demonstrating that love and support are integral to their learning journey.

The second principle, the *what* **of learning**, involves presenting information through various modalities to cater to different learning preferences (UCC, 2021). In a diverse setting where students might be learning in a language that is not their first language, employing multiple representations of content can be especially helpful. Incorporating innovative technologies such as virtual reality (VR) or using varied formats for assessments such as podcasts, videos, and posters can engage different senses and learning styles. By offering diverse methods of teaching and assessing, educators are being loving because they show they care about and can cater for the students' varied needs and learning preferences, enhancing their overall grasp of the material.

The third principle, the *how* **of learning**, focuses on planning and performing tasks effectively. This principle acknowledges that students are unique human beings who all come with different backgrounds and levels of prior knowledge (UCC, 2021). A compassionate approach involves creating opportunities for students to express what they know and guiding them through the learning process with understanding and support. Embracing new technologies and innovative teaching methods with empathy helps students overcome barriers to communication and expression, ensuring that they feel valued and capable. By addressing these needs with care and creativity, educators foster an environment where students can thrive and fully engage in their learning experience.

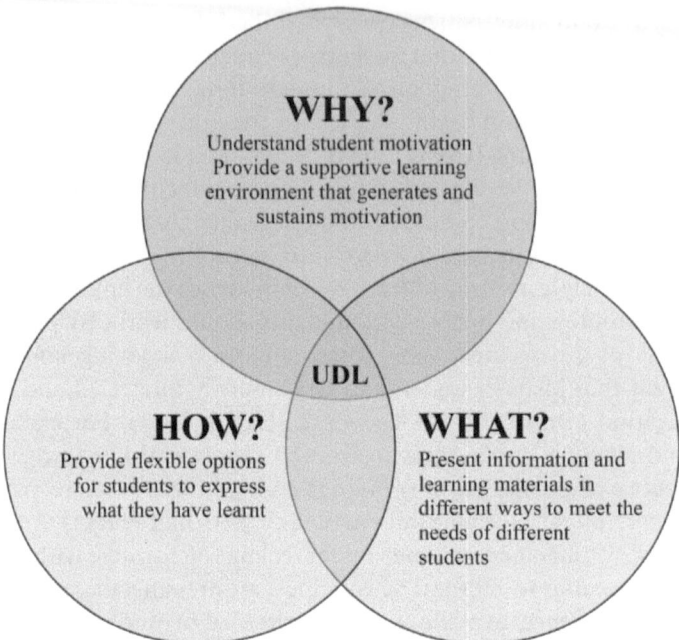

UDL is much more than a box-ticking approach. The principles of UDL are inherently loving because they guide midwifery educators to create an inclusive, nurturing environment and create effective learning materials and activities. UDL has the potential to ensure that students' individual identities, needs, and personal growth are recognised and that this is integral to academic teaching and support.

Learning point: There is not one optimal means of expression for all learners.

REFLECTION FOR MIDWIFERY EDUCATORS

- Do you incorporate the principles of UDL in your teaching and learning practices? If so, how do you ensure that all students have equitable access to the learning experience?
- Can you recall a specific instance when offering different modes of engagement or assessment might have enhanced a student's experience? How might you approach such situations differently in the future?
- What do you see as the primary barriers to implementing a UDL approach in your teaching, and how might these challenges be addressed to better support diverse learners?

Conclusion

At the heart of all the concepts in this chapter lies love, a foundational element in teaching and mentoring. When educators approach their role with genuine care and compassion, they create an environment where students feel supported and valued. This love-driven approach not only helps students navigate the complexities of life but also empowers them to develop resilience, self-awareness, and a commitment to self-care. By promoting these qualities, educators help students build a strong foundation for both their personal and professional lives, ensuring they are not only competent midwives but also well-rounded, emotionally healthy individuals.

References

Adam, A. B., Druye, A. A., Kumi-Kyereme, A., Osman, W., & Alhassan, A. (2021). Nursing and midwifery students' satisfaction with their clinical rotation experience: The role of the clinical learning environment. *Nursing Research and Practice, 2021*, 7258485. https://doi.org/10.1155/2021/7258485

Barrett, A., Burleigh, A., Gillen, P., & Hughes, D. (2023). *#Saynotobullyinginmidwifery*. Association of Radical Midwives.

Carolan-Olah, M., Kruger, G., Walter, R., & Mazzarino, M. (2014). Final year students' experiences of the Bachelor of Midwifery course. *Midwifery, 30*(5), 519–525. https://doi.org/10.1016/j.midw.2013.04.007

CAST. (2024). *Universal design for learning guidelines*. CAST website. https://udl guidelines.cast.org/action-expression/

Elias, M. J. (2016). *4 approaches to building positive community in any classroom. Edutopia.* George Lucas Educational Foundation. https://cms4files1.revize.com/ southlyonschoolsmi/employees/intranet/docs/Classroom%20Culture%20Set-up% 20and%20Management%20Presentation%202018.pdf

Fenwick, J., Cullen, D., Gamble, J., & Sidebotham, M. (2016). Being a young midwifery student: A qualitative exploration. *Midwifery, 39*, 27–34. https://doi.org/10.1016/j. midw.2016.04.010

Francis, R. (2013). *Report of the Mid Staffordshire NHS Foundation Trust public inquiry*. Gov.UK. https://www.gov.uk/government/publications/report-of-the-mid-staffordshire-nhs-foundation-trust-public-inquiry

Gilkison, A., Giddings, L., & Smythe, L. (2016). Real life narratives enhance learning about the 'art and science' of midwifery practice. *Advances in Health Sciences Education: Theory and Practice, 21*(1), 19–32. https://doi.org/10.1007/s10459-015-9607-z

Groothuizen, J. E., Callwood, A., & Gallagher, A. (2018). NHS constitution values for values-based recruitment: A virtue ethics perspective. *Journal of Medical Ethics, 44*(8), 518–523. https://doi.org/10.1136/medethics-2017-104503

Hunter, B., Fenwick, J., Sidebotham, M., & Henley, J. (2019). Midwives in the United Kingdom: Levels of burnout, depression, anxiety and stress and associated predictors. *Midwifery, 79*, 102526. https://doi.org/10.1016/j.midw.2019.08.008

Keller, S., Yule, S., Zagarese, V., & Henrickson Parker, S. (2020). Predictors and triggers of incivility within healthcare teams: A systematic review of the literature. *BMJ Open, 10*(6), e035471. https://doi.org/10.1136/bmjopen-2019-035471

Kuipers, Y. J. (2022). Exploring the uses of virtues in woman-centred care: A quest, synthesis and reflection. *Nursing Philosophy: An International Journal for Healthcare Professionals, 23*(2), e12380. https://doi.org/10.1111/nup.12380

Maslow, A. H. (1954). *Motivation and personality*. Harpers. (p. 236).

Migura, T. (2024). The academisation and Europeanisation of midwifery training in Germany, Austria and Switzerland. *International Journal of Vocational Education Studies, 1*(1), 117–140. https://journals.ub.uni-osnabrueck.de/index.php/ijves/article/view/235

Neiterman, E., Beggs, B., HakemZadeh, F., Zeytinoglu, I., Geraci, J., Oltean, I., Plenderleith, J., & Lobb, D. (2022). "They hold your fate in their hands": Exploring the power dynamic in the midwifery student-preceptor relationship. *Midwifery, 112*, 103430. https://doi.org/10.1016/j.midw.2022.103430

Neiterman, E., HakemZadeh, F., Zeytinoglu, I. U., Kaminska, K., Oltean, I., Plenderleith, J., & Lobb, D. (2024). Navigating interprofessional boundaries: Midwifery students in Canada. *Social Science & Medicine (1982), 341*, 116554. https://doi.org/10.1016/j.socscimed.2023.116554

Nursing and Midwifery Council. (2018). *The code*. https://www.nmc.org.uk/standards/code/

Obara, S., Perry, B., Janzen, K.J., & Edwards, M. (2022). Using arts-based pedagogy to enrich nursing education. *Teaching and Learning in Nursing, 17*(1), 113–120.

Pezaro, S., Clyne, W., Turner, A., Fulton, E. A., & Gerada, C. (2016). 'Midwives Overboard!' Inside their hearts are breaking, their makeup may be flaking but their smile still stays on. *Women and Birth: Journal of the Australian College of Midwives, 29(3)*, e59–e66. https://doi.org/10.1016/j.wombi.2015.10.006

Power, A., & Clews, C. (2015). Values-based recruitment and the NHS Constitution: Making sure student midwives meet the brief. *British Journal of Midwifery, 23*(11), 818–820. https://doi.org/10.12968/bjom.2015.23.11.818

Russell, M. J. (2014). Teaching civility to undergraduate nursing students using a virtue ethics-based curriculum. *The Journal of Nursing Education, 53*(6), 313–319. https://doi.org/10.3928/01484834-20140512-03

Sharif, S. M., Yap, W. S., Fun, W. H., Yoon, E. L., Abd Razak, N. F., Sararaks, S., & Lee, S. W. H. (2021). Midwifery qualification in selected countries: A rapid review. *Nursing Reports, 11*(4), 859–880. https://doi.org/10.3390/nursrep11040080

Spilsbury, K., Thompson, C., Bloor, K., Dale, V., Devi, R., Jackson, C., McCaughan, D., Simpson, A., & Mannion, R. (2022). *Values based recruitment: What works, for whom, why, and in what circumstances? Report*. University of Leeds. https://doi.org/10.48785/100/101

Sweet, L., Bass, J., Sidebotham, M., Fenwick, J., & Graham, K. (2019). Developing reflective capacities in midwifery students: Enhancing learning through reflective writing. *Women and Birth, 32*(2), 119–126.

University College Cork. (2021). *Universal design for learning. General inclusive guidelines*. https://www.ucc.ie/en/udl/general/

Vermeulen, J., Buyl, R., D'haenens, F., Swinnen, E., Stas, L., Gucciardo, L., & Fobelets, M. (2021). Midwifery students' satisfaction with perinatal simulation-based training. *Women and Birth: Journal of the Australian College of Midwives, 34*(6), 554–562. https://doi.org/10.1016/j.wombi.2020.12.006

13

LOVE AND PROFESSIONAL ISSUES IN MIDWIFERY

Diane Ménage

Relationship-based care and professional Issues

Trusting relationships between women and their midwives, or other maternity care professionals, are the mechanisms for safe, high-quality care, promoting women's informed decision making, and increasing service users' satisfaction (Almorbaty et al., 2023; Dahlberg & Aune 2013; O'Brien et al., 2021). It is relational care that allows midwives to practise lovingly or to put it another way: midwifery *is* the relationship (Page, 2016). The evidence points to continuity of carer (CoC) as the best way to promote relational care and shows that it is associated with a range of clinical benefits, including reduced chance of preterm birth and reduced requirements for both epidural in labour and episiotomy (Sandall et al., 2016). In the United Kingdom, plans to implement this model of care were launched separately in Scotland (Scottish Government, 2016), England (NHS England, 2017), and Wales (Welsh Government, 2019). In 2021, guidance was published to deliver CoC in England at full scale (NHS England, 2021). Yet, the following year a report on failings in maternity care at an NHS Trust in England called for suspension of this roll-out unless Trusts could demonstrate that staffing met safe minimum requirements on all shifts (Ockenden, 2022). With a national shortage of midwives, this has meant that for many maternity services the plans to introduce CoC was put on hold. While no country apart from New Zealand has managed to scale up CoC at a national level (Bradford et al., 2022), this is still the gold standard for maternity care. However, relationship-based care is widespread in that midwives in the UK and all over the world build and nurture their relationships with the women and families they care for and recognise this as a fundamental part of care. Indeed, relationships can be built in a very short time, for example, when looking after

DOI: 10.4324/9781032645780-17

a woman in labour, having never met them before. Compassion from midwives in these circumstances is linked to that relationship, and women have reported how the midwife's ability to forge a close and meaningful relationship with them has been a hallmark of compassionate care (Menage et al., 2020).

Many midwives recognise that their practice is driven by a form of love and that their relationships with those they care for are professional yet at the same time close, authentic and genuinely based on care and respect. Yet, the nature of that relationship and the caring, reciprocal feelings that can come with such a close and ongoing relationship (particularly when there is continuity), are not acknowledged by the profession. The paradox is that we know the importance of relationship-based care and yet there has been a failure to address the issues related to successfully forming, maintaining, and ending those relationships. Sometimes this may seem easy and natural, but relationships will be challenging at times. For example, what happens if you do not like the woman that you are looking after? This is a much avoided, taboo subject. For many, it is an uncomfortable subject, yet it is unlikely that we will always like everybody. Most services will accommodate a request for a change of midwife from the service user. However, when it is the midwife who is having difficulties, it usually goes unspoken. Roger Neighbour (2019) has written extensively about patient/relationships in GP practice and his words below acknowledge the issue of not liking or not getting on with some patients:

> We…are human beings too. We have good days and bad days; we have our own personal life stories, our own likes and dislikes, our own attitudes, values, and emotions. It is inevitable that our own personality will sometimes contribute to why we find a particular patient particularly challenging.
>
> *(Neighbour, 2019)*

These words surely ring true for all healthcare practitioners including midwives. Although Neighbour points out that in a relationship the problem is rarely one-sided and that sometimes we ourselves, our personalities and our personal histories are contributing factors. Approaching this problem with love can be helpful in a number of ways. Drawing on Neighbour's work, as well as my own and other's experiences, Box 13.1 provides a reflection and some suggestions on how this may be done.

However very occasionally midwives find themselves faced with a relationship that has broken down and when this happens, it is vital that appropriate support is sought to either rebuild the relationship or end it safely, providing the woman with another midwife that she can build a more constructive relationship with. It is important to do this in a way that minimises any risk to the woman (MacGregor & Smythe, 2014).

Just as it is possible to not like some people, it is also the case that we can like them so much that they feel like *actual* friends and this has the potential to

---

BOX 13.1   RELATIONSHIP DIFFICULTIES: PERSONAL REFLECTION ON YOUR FEELINGS

- It can help you to understand your own part in the difficulty and this requires self-love. See Chapter 9 for more on this. First recognise that you are only human and not perfect. It is important to reflect on why you might feel this way about the person. Do they remind you of somebody or something that you do not like? Could you have a prejudice? Does this person inadvertently 'press your buttons'? Observe the feelings and try to understand them while at the same time recognising your commitment to providing this person with the respect and care that they have a right to.

Two Approaches to Try

- Approaching the person from a place of love can help us to find *something* to like. Commit to finding something about them that you like and start by focussing on that. For example, their accent, their dress sense, or their smile. You will find that doing this will start to counteract negative feelings that you may be having.
- One thing that all types of love have in common is the ability to see another person as unique and special (see Chapter 2). Developing curiosity about a person with the aim of understanding them and their life, even in a very small way, will help us see their specialness and that will help the relationship.

Things to Keep in Mind

- Remember that the love we need to develop in our work is not simply an emotion; it can be a value or principle on which to base our care (see Chapter 1). Love is not easy; it asks a lot of us, but we can use loving intentions to find a way of overcoming negative thoughts and feelings about a person.
- Know that love drives compassion (see Chapter 2), but it is a *practice*, rather than a theory. It will not always come naturally. We don't always get it right, especially with people that we find difficult. We have to *keep practising* it.

---

disrupt objectivity, lead to preferential treatment and emotional dependency. There is a fine line to tread here and the term *professional friend* (Pairman, 2000; Walsh, 1999) best encapsulates this combination of friendliness and professionalism. Qualitative studies have shown that women who are very happy with their care, describe their midwives as being like a friend or family member (Menage et al., 2020) and these relationships are based on equality and inclusiveness (Jepsen et al., 2017). The ability of midwives to provide information in the style of a friend, with respect and compassion rather than from a position of power, is empowering and highly valued by women (Menage et al., 2020).

The midwife feels this friendship connection too and yet they are *professional* friends who need to set and maintain boundaries.

One of the arguments against the idea of love in midwifery is that it risks breaching professional boundaries. This may spring from a misunderstanding around the nature of love in this context and not realising that love is a very broad concept with many different forms, as explained in Chapter 1 of this book. However, in *any* relationship boundaries are needed, whether a relationship with a partner, family member, friend, colleague, or neighbour. The nature of those boundaries will change depending on the nature of the relationship. Boundaries are essential for healthy relationships and therefore they are a vital aspect of loving midwifery care. Maintaining boundaries in any relationship can be tricky at times and in relationships with the women and families we care for there are times when clear guidance is needed. One such time is when discharging women from midwifery care.

In relationship-based midwifery care both parties know that the relationship is time-limited. Yet, the end of the relationship, at the end of the care episode or on discharge from midwifery care, is hardly ever discussed in our profession. Although such endings happen often in a midwifery career, it can be an emotional time, particularly when CoC has led to close relationships. Yet, we know little about how midwives and women navigate this ending because there is no acknowledgement of how authentic feelings of caring and love can be part of this relationship, therefore there has not been much scope to explore it. This is an omission and going forward we need more honesty about how relationship-based care is about a *relationship*, and more research on how that relationship develops and how it either changes or ends following discharge from maternity services. This could help to provide professional guidance that is fit for purpose. The following section further discusses the example of the women/midwife relationship after discharge from care and takes a closer look at current guidance on professional boundaries.

Love and professional boundaries

Within a CoC model, discharging a woman from care can be a very happy and positive time but it can also bring feelings of sadness for the woman and the midwife. Some women may seek to continue the relationship as friends and some midwives may see this as a useful way of stepping down the relationship while still keeping in touch. The words of individual midwives in Box 13.2 are testimony to this. It is time to acknowledge these very real feelings and prepare student midwives, as part of their pre-registration education programmes, to not just build relationships lovingly with women and families but also to be able to bring them to an end in a way that works for everyone concerned.

Perhaps there are ways in which the relationship can continue on a different level after care has finished. When women and families have gone through such

---

**BOX 13.2   PROFESSIONAL BOUNDARIES: MIDWIVES'
EXPERIENCES AFTER DISCHARGE**

As a midwife providing continuity of care, I grew very close to the women and families that I was working with. For many of them that relationship started when they were only a few weeks into their pregnancy, and they were only discharged when the baby was four to six weeks old. I looked after some of these women for several pregnancies and felt inextricably linked with them forever. Discharges could be emotional. Women often wanted to keep in touch. I genuinely cared for these women but I knew the relationship had to change at that point. But I always remembered their baby's first birthday and sent a card or a message, and I know that meant a lot to them. Women sometimes got in touch about things many months after they had been discharged. That can be difficult to manage. Emma, Midwife UK.

18 years down the line I have contact with clients. Only yesterday I met up with a client and her daughter (7 yrs) for a coffee and a catch-up. Jane, Former Independent Midwife UK.

I really valued the privilege of caring for women and their families in a relational model of care here in New Zealand and I have maintained contact with some. However, I do feel that this is best framed within the context of a professional relationship. I have seen things go horribly wrong between women and midwives where dependency becomes an issue, both co-dependency and one sided. It's important to have this subject embedded in midwifery education. I agree that we need to accept that social media is an integral part of life in 2024 but I would also suggest that its use in a practice context has some potential fishhooks that should be explored, within a supportive learning context. It's not about trying to silo or stymie relationships but about being mindful. Lorna, Midwife New Zealand.

I do love the women I care for. Obviously, it's not the same as how I love my partner or my family...but definitely, I do. Saying a final goodbye to people can be so hard. As a bereavement midwife, I just don't discharge anyone, even though they may be medically discharged, they may still need emotional support. So, regarding support, I don't discharge them because I would *always* talk to them. Sarah, Bereavement Midwife, UK.

---

life-changing experiences, they may want to talk to one of the few people who was there with them. For example, bereavement midwife Sarah (Box 13.2) has developed her own practice regarding discharging women which works for her and those she has cared for. This is not catered for in current guidance.

There is clearly a need for up-to-date guidance to help midwives navigate the challenges and dilemmas that can occur in these relationships. Professional guidance varies widely throughout the world. In the UK, the Nursing and Midwifery Council [NMC] (2019a) Code of Practice states that nurses and midwives must

> stay objective and have clear professional boundaries at all times with people in your care (including those who have been in your care in the past), their families and carers.
>
> *(Paragraph 20.6)*

How should we interpret this extremely broad statement? One starting place is understanding what professional boundaries are. But this is far from straightforward. It is very difficult to find any definitions on what professional boundaries are in relation to midwifery. One exception is the guidance on using social media in which the NMC (n.d.) say:

> Nurses, midwives, and nursing associates should not use social networks to build or pursue relationships with patients and service users as this can blur important professional boundaries.

There is a clear directive on social media use here but once again no definition or explanation of what professional boundaries are. However, anecdotally, many midwives do communicate with service users on social media, suggesting that more detailed guidance and rationale is needed on this.

In other countries, there may be more or less explanation of what constitutes professional boundaries. In 2018, the Nursing and Midwifery Board in Australia (NMBA) stated that:

> Professional boundaries allow midwives, the woman and the woman's nominated partners, family and friends, to engage safely and effectively in professional relationships, including where care involves personal and/or intimate contact. In order to maintain professional boundaries, there is a start and end point to the professional relationship, and it is integral to the midwife-woman professional relationship. Adhering to professional boundaries promotes woman-centred practice and protects both parties.
>
> *(NMBA Code of Conduct, Principle 4.1)*

The NMBA also introduces the concept of the therapeutic relationship, a concept which is surely key to relationship-based care, aspects of which reflect the *professional friend* discussed earlier. They go on to define the nature of the therapeutic relationship and provide more detailed information on the sorts of behaviours that would breach professional boundaries (NMBA, 2018). The NMBA Code of Conduct provides significantly more guidance than the NMC offers in the UK. Nevertheless, midwifery standards and guidance on this matter seem to be contradictory. On the one hand, midwives should develop good relationships with women and families based on trust, respect, and caring. Yet, on the other hand, following discharge they should behave as if there is no relationship.

The NMBA's Code of Conduct is very clear about the woman/midwife relationship having a start and end point, but in the past midwives were part of, and well known within, the communities they served. In many rural parts of the developing world today, it is likely that the midwife is already known to the women as a friend, neighbour, or relative. In such communities, the woman–midwife relationship weaves in and out of kinship and friend relationships, seemingly with ease. Indie's words in Box 13.3 describe how this works in rural Ethiopia. What Indie describes may seem a very long way from the sort of midwifery practised in most modern maternity facilities. Nevertheless, many midwives working in modern maternity units, when pregnant themselves, seek out a midwife colleague they know well and ask them to be their midwife. CoC models can and do resemble this sort of close midwife/woman relationship, fostering feelings of connectedness and familiarity which extend well beyond clinical care (Kelly et al., 2014).

Indie's words are a testimony to the very different practices regarding relationships in midwifery, which might be considered problematic in many other parts of the world. However, there may be something to learn from this: that women and midwives are capable of navigating changing relationships.

In the UK, medical defence barristers have noted that most breaches of professional boundaries in the healthcare sector are associated with "improper

---

BOX 13.3 MIDWIVES AND WOMEN NAVIGATING RELATIONSHIPS IN ETHIOPIA

It is expected that midwives at the clinic will look after their female relatives and their neighbours. I can say with absolute confidence that no one thinks that this is remotely unusual or unwise. There is no sense of conflict of interest when looking after friends, family (one of the traditional midwives was midwife to her own mother), co-workers or neighbours. But in a rural community that's largely closed off, in the sense that the same families have lived here for generations and by tribe or blood or marriage, pretty much everyone is related, it would be almost impossible to have it otherwise. My experience is that both women and midwives are more than capable of navigating relationships that require different boundaries in different circumstances. Indie, midwife, researcher, and anthropologist with experience of practising in rural Ethiopia relationships," allegations of sexual impropriety, financial conflicts of interest, and psychological and physical harm (McCaffrey, 2023). These are extremely serious breaches that women must be protected from. Nevertheless, it should be possible to have professional guidance which acknowledges the feelings of genuine caring in woman–midwife relationships, and yet still promote safe boundaries for women and midwives. In addition, opportunities to explore these issues within pre-registration midwifery programmes may help to prepare midwives with some of the skills needed to navigate issues around building and ending relationships.

Midwifery research as a form of love

The Lancet Series definition of midwifery states that it is "skilled, knowledgeable and compassionate care" for childbearing women and families across the childbirth continuum (Renfrew et al., 2014, p. 1130). A strong midwifery profession is built on a body of knowledge; that knowledge is developed through experience and clinical expertise, but it must also come from empirical research. Such knowledge is the basis of safe, evidence-based practice and without midwifery research we do not have a credible profession. As midwives, we have a professional duty to critically analyse, share, and apply research findings and to base our practice on best available evidence (NMC, 2019b) and we also have a role in advancing midwifery knowledge (International Confederation of Midwives [ICM], 2023).

We live in an age when almost everybody turns to the internet to get their questions answered, it has never been more important to remind ourselves that all information is not equal. To understand what constitutes current best evidence and what does not, midwives need to differentiate between research-based evidence and opinion, journalism, and misinformation. The use of Artificial Intelligence (AI) will not necessarily be able to help with this. While it certainly has a growing role in healthcare, AI platforms and chatbots such as ChatGPT are not well-positioned to distinguish between what is factually correct and what is not (Meyrowitsch et al., 2023).

If we want to provide the best care, it is vital to keep asking questions about what this entails. Both quantitative and qualitative research is needed to answer these questions; which form is used will depend on the research question. Quantitative research is required if we want to measure cause and effect with measurable outcomes, e.g., if we want to know if a new breastfeeding preparation class increases breastfeeding initiation and continuation. But if we want to understand why women stop breastfeeding after only a short time, we need qualitative research to explore these women's experiences, thoughts, and feelings. Research questions spring from our own curiosity but perhaps the most important questions come from seeing that something is not right and trying to find out how it can best be improved.

Research also gives voice to those who use maternity services and listening to and seeking to understand women's experiences of care is a *loving* thing to do. Because when we care about somebody, we want the best for them and if we notice that they are having difficulties (of any sort) we want to understand these.

It is perhaps when midwives and women work together to conduct research that it can be most beneficial. Collaborative research, in which studies are conceptualised and co-created, work by bringing together researchers and service users to facilitate improvements in services. By researching *with* the communities that receive maternity services, the resulting evidence has the potential to make an impact in the real world (Greenhalgh et al., 2016). In this way *co-creation* spans both research and service improvement. For example, Dyson et al. (2023) wanted to tackle problems with communication between women and midwives about alcohol use in pregnancy. Barriers to open and honest communication had already been identified through previous studies. But what the researchers did was to use a co-creative approach, in which women whose babies had Fetal Alcohol Spectrum Disorder, came together with midwives to find ways of reducing these barriers and improving conversations about alcohol in pregnancy.

The role of compassion in scientific inquiry is not a new idea. It was something that Mahatma Gandhi was interested in, and the 14th Dalai Lama has actively engaged with scientists in fields such as neuroscience and psychology to explore how compassion can be understood and cultivated, demonstrating a clear link between a love for humanity and research. In maternity care we can see how the impetus for conducting a study may come from noticing suffering (such as poor maternal and neonatal outcomes) and asking important questions about how such suffering can be reduced. It could be a response to maternal mortality statistics for example. It is known that in the UK maternal mortality is higher in Black and Asian women (Felker et al., 2024) and research into the possible reasons for this is vital, so that this can be reduced.

Noticing suffering might also come from something observed in practice. For example, through her work Jenny Patterson became aware of the growing number of women who developed birth trauma following childbirth. Through initial research, Patterson identified that the woman/midwife interaction was the strongest predictor of birth trauma and then had a question: how did women who developed birth trauma, experience their interactions with midwives? She conducted a study aimed at understanding how women who develop birth trauma post childbirth, *and* midwives, experience their interactions and what this means to them (Patterson et al., 2019). There are parallels between this process and the process of compassion; it clearly involved noticing suffering and trying to respond in a way that would achieve greater insights into the problem, building understanding which could eventually lead to a reduction in suffering.

For many midwives, it is perhaps easier to see loving midwifery practice as only relevant to aspects of clinical practice. Unfortunately, midwifery research can be thought of as being rather dry, boring, and even irrelevant (Corr, 2018). This needs to change. Therefore, it is important that the topic is taught well in undergraduate programmes, and this includes making clear links between evidence-based practice and research; introducing students to passionate midwifery researchers and their work; explaining how research is pivotal for the profession and is actually a part of *loving* midwifery practice.

Healing toxic maternity cultures with love

In many parts of the world, midwives work in problematic maternity systems that are under-resourced, poorly led, and frequently do not meet the needs of service users. There is a lot at stake in maternity care; the consequences of poor outcomes are devastating and far reaching. When things go wrong, understandably the families involved want to know how and why. The processes used to provide these answers are important because this can lead to better understanding and real learning, which can lead to improved practice. In order to achieve this, an open, honest, caring culture is required. Maternity cultures which are rooted in fear and blame block this and lead to reluctance to admit mistakes and cover-ups. A catalogue of investigations and reports in maternity care in the UK over recent years has found that learning lessons from mistakes is often lacking. It is evident that the culture of maternity care is resistant to change. The Ockenden Report highlighted how poor communication and lack of collaboration between different healthcare professionals had a significant impact on the quality of care to mothers and babies (Ockenden, 2022). Inability to share important information in a timely, effective manner led to mismanagement of complications, in some cases with tragic outcomes. The report emphasised the need to improve teamwork and communication between doctors and midwives. So, what is going wrong here?

Doctors and midwives have distinct roles and undergo different education and training. Nevertheless, a safe maternity care service requires both. Women want safe, high-quality maternity care and this should be provided by midwives and sometimes doctors, as and when appropriate to their needs. The key thing to remember here is that to those receiving maternity care it is *all one service*. Many maternity units do reflect this and manage to build great teams who communicate well. If you have worked in a service like that (and I have), you will know how good this is for the women and their families as well as for the staff. But if you have worked in a service that is marred by power differentials and hierarchy, where big egos, chips on shoulders, an *us* and *them* culture (Lephard, 2024) or *othering* prevails (and I have witnessed this too), you will recognise ways in which it detracts from good care, and you will know how unpleasant it is to work in. What is lacking in these services is respect, trust, and kindness, or to put it another way, the will to work *lovingly* with all our colleagues. Service-users notice when there is a problem between staff, and they hate it. A qualitative study by Watson et al. (2016) found women clearly noticed when there was tension and conflict between midwives and doctors and found it distressing. That is not to say that professionals cannot disagree, but it is about how they manage disagreements. However, it is not just about midwives and doctors. There can be a hierarchy between junior and senior midwives which leads to dysfunctional working relationships in which there is a fear to speak up, even when it is about poor care or safety concerns (Elliott-Mainwaring, 2021). The bullying and disrespect of both midwives and doctors working in obstetrics is well documented (Royal College of Obstetrics and Gynaecology [RCOG] & Royal College of Midwives [RCM], 2021) and it is harmful to the practitioners and those they are caring for.

Poor relationships between maternity staff create dangerous, toxic working environments and unsafe care. This is one of the leading professional issues facing midwives right now. Nobody is a winner when there is conflict between those working within the same service. What is more, in midwifery there can be a tendency for midwives addressing the problems around the medicalisation of childbirth, being viewed as anti-doctor. Midwives have rightly tried to occupy their place as experts in physiological birth, yet for some reason, it has been accompanied by the false premise that midwives think medical intervention is wrong. The midwife's role in understanding and supporting the physiological processes of birth was never about physiological birth *versus* medicalised birth. All women need a midwife, and some women will need a doctor too, such as when complications arise or if the woman wants or needs something outside the midwife's sphere of practice. Contrary to what the media might portray, the vast majority of midwives are well aware that obstetrics is a vital part of maternity care and when there are serious complications, it is lifesaving. But unfortunately, midwives and doctors are being portrayed as adversaries.

It does not have to be like this. The solution is to move away from polarised ideologies around birth, e.g., physiological birth versus medicalisation of childbirth and build teams that understand the value of everyone in the maternity team. This means respecting midwives' expertise *and* that of the other clinicians who provide maternity care and working collaboratively to avoid interventions that are *too much too soon* or *too little too late* (Downe et al., 2020).

Using love as an underpinning value would achieve this. There are those who will read this and think that this is a passive response, in which midwives will lose their identity and power, but it is far from it. This approach takes strength. Midwives who have a strong professional identity and are confident in their role, knowledge, and skills, and have emotional intelligence can and do work *respectfully as equals* within the multidisciplinary team, providing supportive role models for student midwives and newly qualified midwives. But, in order to maintain this, a number of things need to be in place. The profession urgently needs to concentrate efforts on strong midwifery leadership, eradicating an *us* and *them* culture and improving working relationships in maternity care as outlined in Box 13.4.

BOX 13.4   STRATEGIES FOR HEALING TOXIC MATERNITY CULTURES

1) Build a strong midwifery profession

For this, we need to continually develop the body of knowledge that underpins midwifery practice and education (see midwifery research from a place of love earlier in this chapter). If we are competent and confident in our knowledge and skills, we can rightly claim our place as experts in physiological pregnancy, birth, and the postpartum period. But there are always (at least) two experts making decisions, one is the midwife, and one is the woman. When there are complications or when women have particular preferences, there will be an obstetrician and/or anaesthetist and/or a paediatrician too and midwives can lovingly lead the way, expecting and demonstrating collaborative, respectful team working.

2) Eradicating *us* and *them* within maternity teams.

This does not mean that midwives will lose their identity. Practitioners in a strong profession can be confident and comfortable in their role without feeling threatened by other disciplines. Our future as a profession is in developing ourselves, respecting ourselves and others, not berating others. Midwives and other maternity care professionals are usually incredibly good at making people feel welcome and included but there is always a need to look out for, and guard against, that *othering* as described in Chapter 1.

3) More emphasis on positive working relationships in pre-registration education and training

This requires a focus on building emotional intelligence, and activities that develop listening skills, clear communication, and assertiveness. This means that there needs to be much more emphasis on learning and practising these techniques in a safe, confidential learning space with skilled support. For example, role-playing different clinical scenarios, which may require negotiation such as having difficult conversations with other members of the team and learning how to maintain personal and professional boundaries. Some universities use actors and/or trained service users to facilitate role play, helping students to: see a situation from the other's perspective; explore their own emotional responses in different scenarios; and try out different strategies for dealing with challenging situations. Much can be achieved through interprofessional education, which should not be a tick box exercise but a real opportunity to learn about each other's roles. Learning with other care professionals improves understanding about each other's roles (Choudhury et al., 2020) and therefore has the potential to promote mutual respect and better communication.

Reflections and conclusions

Throughout this book, many different ways have been presented in which love can be seen as a legitimate part of midwifery, and midwifery can be seen as an expression of love. This chapter has presented new ideas and perspectives on the need for love in our profession and suggested ways in which love can help to build a strong, sustainable profession. It has also identified ways in which the profession needs to adapt in order to support loving practice. Cultures do not change quickly but they can change one person at a time. A profession is made up of people and each one can make a difference. If enough of those people bring love to their work and their working relationships, we will have a loving profession.

As you come to the end of this chapter on Love and Professional Issues, you are invited to reflect on what you have read. Which of the four professional issues discussed (relationship-based care, boundaries, research, and healing toxic maternity cultures) resonated with you most? Do you think that practising lovingly is unprofessional or do you think that bringing love into your work is perfectly compatible with professionalism? It is hoped that the chapter has helped you to reflect on how you can build on these new perspectives to make your own professional practice more rewarding and meaningful.

How midwives harness and use their love for their profession, those they care for, their colleagues and for themselves is very individual. It should be seen as something that is ongoing, a strong motivator for our development and a powerful lens with which to consider our work and our profession. Using love as a value on which to base our practice, as described in Chapter 1, can assist us with difficult decisions about what is important, helping us to keep the love we have for our work at the forefront of what we do.

References

Almorbaty, H., Ebert, L., Dowse, E., & Chan, S. W. (2023). An integrative review of supportive relationships between child-bearing women and midwives. *Nursing open*, *10*(3), 1327–1339. https://doi.org/10.1002/nop2.1447

Bradford, B. F., Wilson, A. N., Portela, A., McConville, F., Fernandez Turienzo, C., & Homer, C. S. E. (2022). Midwifery continuity of care: A scoping review of where, how, by whom and for whom?. *PLOS Global Public Health*, *2*(10), e0000935. https://doi.org/10.1371/journal.pgph.0000935

Choudhury, R. I., Salam, M. A. U., Mathur, J., & Choudhury, S. R. (2020). How inter-professional education could benefit the future of healthcare - Medical students' perspective. *BMC Medical Education*, *20*(1). https://doi.org/10.1186/s12909-020-02170-w

Corr, A. (2018). "No offence, it's just that research is boring": The trials and tribulations of the midwifery research educator. *British Journal of Midwifery*, *26*(7), 470–474. https://doi.org/10.12968/bjom.2018.26.7.470

Dahlberg, U., & Aune, I. (2013). The woman's birth experience—The effect of interpersonal relationships and continuity of care. *Midwifery*, *29*(4), 407–415. https://doi.org/10.1016/j.midw.2012.09.006

Downe, S., Calleja Agius, J., Balaam, M. C., & Frith, L. (2020). Understanding childbirth as a complex salutogenic phenomenon: *The EU COST BIRTH action special collection*. *PloS One*, *15*(8), e0236722. https://doi.org/10.1371/journal.pone.0236722

Dyson, J., Onukwugha, F., Howlett, H., Combe, K., Catterick, M., & Smith, L. (2023). Midwives and service users' perspectives on implementing a dialogue about alcohol use in antenatal care: A qualitative study. *Journal of Advanced Nursing*, *79*(8), 2955–2966. https://doi.org/10.1111/jan.15622

Elliott-Mainwaring, H. (2021). How do power and hierarchy influence staff safety in maternity services? *British Journal of Midwifery*, *29*(8), 430–439. https://doi.org/10.12968/bjom.2021.29.8.430

Greenhalgh, T., Jackson, C., Shaw, S., & Janamian, T. (2016). Achieving research impact through co-creation in community-based health services: Literature review and case study. *The Milbank quarterly*, *94*(2), 392–429. https://doi.org/10.1111/1468-0009.12197

Jepsen, I., Mark, E., Foureur, M., Nøhr, E. A., & Sørensen, E. E. (2017). A qualitative study of how caseload midwifery is experienced by couples in Denmark. *Women and birth: journal of the Australian College of Midwives*, *30*(1), e61–e69. https://doi.org/10.1016/j.wombi.2016.09.003

International Confederation of Midwives. (2023). *Role of the midwife in research*. https://internationalmidwives.org/resources/role-of-the-midwife-in-research/

Kelly, J., West, R., Gamble, J., Sidebotham, M., Carson, V., & Duffy, E. (2014). 'She knows how we feel': Australian aboriginal and Torres Strait Islander childbearing women's experience of continuity of care with an Australian aboriginal and Torres Strait Islander midwifery student. *Women and Birth: Journal of the Australian College of Midwives*, *27*(3), 157–162. https://doi.org/10.1016/j.wombi.2014.06.002

Lephard, E. (2024). No more 'Us' and 'Them'. *The Practising Midwife*, *27*(5), 29–31. https://doi.org/10.55975/CZMU3005

Felker, A., Patel, R., Kotnis, R, Kenyon, S., & Knight, M. (Eds.) (2024). *Saving lives, improving mothers' care: Lessons learned to inform maternity care from the UK and Ireland confidential enquiries into maternal deaths and morbidity 2020-22*. MBRRACE-UK. Oxford: National Perinatal Epidemiology Unit, University of Oxford. https://www.npeu.ox.ac.uk/mbrrace-uk/reports/maternal-reports/maternal-report-2020-2022

MacGregor, D., & Smythe, L. (2014). When the midwife-woman partnership breaks down – Principles for ending the relationship. *New Zealand College of Midwives Journal*, *49*, 11–16. https://www.midwife.org.nz/wp-content/uploads/2018/12/Jnl-49-art-2-When-the-midwife-woman-partnership.pdf

McCaffrey, S. (2023, Aug 14). *Maintaining professional boundaries for doctors – A cautionary tale*. https://stephenmccaffreybarrister.com/?s=professional+boundaries

Menage, D., Bailey, E., Lees, S., & Coad, J. (2020). Women's lived experience of compassionate midwifery: Human and professional. *Midwifery*, *85*, 102662. https://doi.org/10.1016/j.midw.2020.102662

Meyrowitsch, D. W., Jensen, A. K., Sørensen, J. B., & Varga, T. V. (2023). AI chatbots and (mis)information in public health: Impact on vulnerable communities. *Frontiers in public health*, *11*, 1226776. https://doi.org/10.3389/fpubh.2023.1226776

Neighbour, R. (2019), Challenging consultations. *InnovAiT*, *12*(1), 24–29. https://doi. org/10.1177/1755738018800356

NHS England. (2017). *Implementing better births: Continuity of carer. Five year forward view*. NHS England. https://www.england.nhs.uk/wp-content/uploads/2017/12/ implementing-better-births.pdf

NHS England. (2021). *Delivering midwifery continuity of carer at full scale: Guidance on planning, implementation and monitoring 2021/22*. NHS England. https://www. england.nhs.uk/publication/delivering-midwifery-continuity-of-carer-at-full-scale- guidance-21-22/

Nursing and Midwifery Board of Australia. (2018). *Code of conduct*. https://www. nursingmidwiferyboard.gov.au/Codes-Guidelines-Statements/Professional-standards. aspx

Nursing and Midwifery Council. (2019a). *The code. Professional standards of practice and behaviour for nurses, midwives and nursing associates*. Nursing and Midwifery Council. https://www.nmc.org.uk/standards/code/

Nursing and Midwifery Council. (2019b). *Standards of proficiency for midwives*. https:// www.nmc.org.uk/standards/standards-for-midwives/standards-of-proficiency- for-midwives/

Nursing and Midwifery Council. (n.d.). *Social media guidance*. Nursing and Midwifery Council. www.nmc.org.uk/standards/guidance/social-media-guidance/

O'Brien, D., Butler, M. M., & Casey, M. (2021). The importance of nurturing trusting relationships to embed shared decision-making during pregnancy and childbirth. *Midwifery*, *98*, 102987. https://doi.org/10.1016/j.midw.2021.102987

Ockenden, D. (2022). *Final report of the Ockenden review. Findings, conclusions and essential actions from the independent review of maternity services at the Shrewsbury and Telford Hospital NHS Trust*. Department of Health and Social Care. https:// www.gov.uk/government/publications/final-report-of-the-ockenden-review

Page, L. (2016). Midwifery: The relationship that heals. *Practising Midwife*, *19*(5), 6. https://www.all4maternity.com/viewpoint-midwifery-relationship-heals/

Pairman, S. (2000) Women-centred midwifery: Partnerships or professional friend- ships? In M. Kirkham (Ed). *The midwife-mother relationship*. (pp. 207–226). Macmillan Press Ltd.

Patterson, J., Hollins Martin, C. J., & Karatzias, T. (2019). Disempowered midwives and traumatised women: Exploring the parallel processes of care provider interaction that contribute to women developing Post Traumatic Stress Disorder (PTSD) post childbirth. *Midwifery*, *76*, 21–35. https://doi.org/10.1016/j.midw.2019.05.010

Renfrew, M. J., McFadden, A., Bastos, M. H., Campbell, J., Channon, A. A., Cheung, N. F., Silva, D. R., Downe, S., Kennedy, H. P., Malata, A., McCormick, F., Wick, L., & Declercq, E. (2014). Midwifery and quality care: Findings from a new evidence- informed framework for maternal and newborn care. *Lancet (London, England)*, *384*(9948), 1129–1145. https://doi.org/10.1016/S0140-6736(14)60789-3

Royal College of Obstetrics and Gynaecology & Royal College of Midwives. (2021). *Joint statement on undermining and bullying in the workplace*. https://www.rcog.org. uk/careers-and-training/starting-your-og-career/workforce/improving-workplace- behaviours/rcog-and-rcm-joint-statement-on-undermining-and-bullying-in- the-workplace/

Sandall, J., Soltani, H., Gates, S., Shennan, A., & Devane, D. (2016). Midwife-led con- tinuity models versus other models of care for childbearing women. *The Cochrane database of systematic reviews*, *4*(4), CD004667. https://doi.org/10.1002/14651858. CD004667.pub5

Scottish Government. (2016). *The best start: five year plan for maternity and neonatal care*. Scottish Government. https://www.gov.scot/publications/best-start-five-year-forward-plan-maternity-neonatal-care-scotland/pages/8/

Walsh D. (1999). An ethnographic study of women's experience of partnership caseload midwifery practice: The professional as a friend. *Midwifery*, *15*(3), 165–176. https://doi.org/10.1016/s0266-6138(99)90061-x

Watson, B. M., Heatley, M. L., Gallois, C., & Kruske, S. (2016). The importance of effective communication in interprofessional practice: Perspectives of maternity clinicians. *Health Communication*, *31*(4), 400–407. https://doi.org/10.1080/10410236. 2014.960992

Welsh Government. (2019). Maternity care in Wales – A five-year vision for the future (2019–2014). *Welsh Government*. https://www.gov.wales/sites/default/files/publications/2019-06/maternity-care-in-wales-a-five-year-vision-for-the-future-2019-2024.pdf

CONCLUSION

Strength, growth, and transformation

Diane Ménage and Jenny Patterson

At the start of this book, we explained how, up until now, there had been little serious exploration of love in relation to midwifery practice. We hope that this book has begun to rectify this by starting a conversation about love. Yet, it is just the beginning; our purpose now is to ensure that the conversation continues to grow and develop.

The individual chapters have, in very different ways, considered various aspects of love and their applicability within midwifery. The chapters in Part I addressed the questions: what is love and why do we need to talk about it in maternity care? It delved into love at the very start of life and why those very first connections between a baby and their mother or other primary carer, in the time following birth, are so important. It also explored why there is a pressing need to talk about love at this moment in time and argues that love is part of reimagining a humanised maternity care system. Part II used Chapman's five love languages as a way of approaching some of the manifestations of love in midwifery practice, with chapters on love as touch, acts, words, time, and gift. Part III tackled professional issues with chapters on love for self, for colleagues, and love in leadership and education. The final chapter took a closer look at four specific professional issues (relationships, boundaries, research, and culture change). Together, these three parts of the book articulate a compelling vision of love as the foundation of midwifery practice, and one which is particularly needed now during the troubling times in maternity services that many of the chapters referred to. The book has highlighted the importance of seeing each person as unique, prioritising individualised care that honours the specialness and worth of every human being. This perspective fosters deep

DOI: 10.4324/9781032645780-18

connections and relationships that transcend barriers and has the potential to create an inclusive environment.

The diamond as a representation of love

In Chapter 2, love was described as intentional, relational energy and was likened to a multifaceted diamond; this image was the inspiration for the book's cover. Love is often only thought of in a very narrow way, but love is a big concept and, like a cut diamond with many facets, love can be expressed and lived out in a multitude of ways. Love (like a diamond) is a beautiful thing yet is more than this; it is a thing of substance. One of the themes through this book is that love is not the soft, fluffy feeling that popular culture would have us believe. A diamond is one of the hardest and strongest substances on earth and love too is extremely strong. It is also hard. By that we mean that it is resilient and durable, but also that it is hard because it is not the easy option. Love can be very challenging at times, but it is *always* a thing of meaning and value.

There is much talk of *hard* and *soft* skills in healthcare, with compassion, communication, integrity, and even leadership (all skills necessary when providing loving care) seen as soft skills. But this term is inadequate and misleading because the word soft can imply that something is weak, feeble, or unsubstantial (Parlamis & Monnot, 2019). There is nothing soft about these so-called soft skills (Goldman & Wong, 2020), yet they are not the only skills needed. Loving midwifery care demands knowledge, practical skills, and appropriate behaviour. Women and families need to be lovingly cared for by midwives who: understand physiology, practise evidence-based care, have clinical expertise, *and* emotional intelligence. Loving midwifery care is the *whole package*. No midwife can get this right all the time but many midwives, all over the world, find it meaningful to try to work towards it every day. So what is loving midwifery? It is the midwife who works collaboratively with others for the best outcomes for the women and babies. It is the midwife educator you loved to learn from as a student. It is the leader who sees your worth and encourages you. It is the midwife who speaks up for those without a voice. It is the midwife who speaks up for herself. It is the midwife who *loves* midwifery and is not going to let anyone or anything take that away. It is the midwife who "sort of shines" (Byrom & Downe, 2010); who (like a diamond) attracts the light and reflects it back to others. It is the midwife who is always a work in progress (because she is only human) but who has the will to try to do better because, deep inside, she is driven by the most powerful thing in the world – love. Perhaps that midwife is you?

In Chapter 1, it was argued that love is not something out there; it is already within us. Moreover, love is not merely an emotion but a verb, manifesting in our actions and choices. Midwifery can be seen as an ongoing practice of love, where continuous learning, reflection, and the honing of skills become integral to physically and psychologically safe care. This dedication to excellence in practice ensures that love remains visible in every interaction, from providing care to a woman in labour to advocating for systemic change; from upholding women's reproductive rights to making a drink for colleagues. It is an approach to all these things and more.

Love is about caring. If deep down you care, then you love. Loving care is curious and kind and it helps us to really listen to others. But it also asks a lot of us. It takes courage, vulnerability, and a commitment to continually develop the knowledge and skills we need in midwifery. Love powers that drive to improve both our clinical skills and relationship-building skills and use them together.

Although love is often thought of in spiritual terms and is an aspect of many of the world's religions, it is accessible to all. Love can be held as a core value by midwives of all religions and midwives of none. Everyone's love counts and can shape the way care is delivered. Throughout this book, we have examined how love grounds and enables practitioners but also acts as a guiding force in their decision-making processes. Using love as an underpinning value helps midwives ask and find answers to pivotal questions such as:

What am I here for?
What do I think is important?
What is the loving thing to do now?

Love embodies a commitment to doing what you think is right. It compels us to act ethically and to stand up against inequalities that threaten the dignity of individuals. It intertwines with justice, fairness, and respect, urging us to be advocates for women, colleagues, and ourselves.

Like a diamond, love finds the light and works with it, reflecting that light back, even when circumstances seem very dark. There has never been a time when we have needed love more than now. In the difficult culture and environment experienced by midwives within many maternity settings, it can sometimes seem impossible to see the light. This is when we need love most, because love can be the means of climbing out of that dark place. Love is hopeful and forward-looking and there is evidence that midwives and other maternity care professionals and champions are lovingly working towards the light. Below are some examples of hopeful and forward-looking initiatives.

- **Team Initiatives**
  Many loving team initiatives have been brought to our attention during the course of editing this book, here is just one of them: midwife Emily Patterson had the idea to set up a walking group at South Warwickshire Hospital, England. The group provides opportunities for midwives to get together socially, get some fresh air and exercise and to talk to each other. The walks

provide the space to build supportive relationships and create bonds outside of the hospital setting, and this in turn builds better working relationships.

- **A Local Initiative**
  The Raham Project has been set up by a UK midwife Faiza Rehmen to support women and families from diverse ethnic backgrounds. Driven by Faiza's passion for all things midwifery, she wanted to address the disparity in health outcomes for ethnic minority mothers as well as mothers and babies. The support is focussed around pregnancy, childbirth, and the postpartum period, with an emphasis on maintaining and improving maternal mental wellbeing. The support includes informational support, emotional support, advocacy and a listening session (Raham Project, 2024).

- **A National Initiative**
  Juliet Rayment has embarked on a project funded by The Point of Care Foundation.

  Referrals to the Nursing and Midwifery Council are most often related to patients and families reporting their experiences of lack of kindness, compassion or communication. By facilitating conversations between members of the public, regulators, midwives and student midwives, Juliet is exploring ways that regulators could support positive relationships in maternity care (Point of Care Foundation, 2024).

- **An International Initiative**
  Professor of midwifery Yvonne Kuipers and colleagues set up the *All-you-need-to-know-about-continuity-of-carer* newsletter. It is a successful initiative, spreading positivity about continuity of midwifery carer and relational care. It reaches out to an interested international audience, building continuity of carer capacity and increasing positive attitudes. By delivering uplifting stories in a midwifery culture and using positive language and images, the newsletter is a space where ideas flourish and connections deepen. The vast increase in number of readers from an initial 300 growing to 6000 within less than a year, across Europe, Australia, Asia, and Northern America, shows how impactful and sparking the messages are. Each newsletter brings fresh perspectives that resonate with the midwifery community and celebrate continuity of carer achievements. The initiative is building a network of informed and motivated individuals, amplifying positivity about continuity of carer (Kuipers et al., 2025).

The tree as a representation of love in midwifery

While the diamond is a powerful symbol to help understand some of the characteristics of love, it does not show us love within a whole system. As a way of bringing together the different aspects of love in midwifery which have been developed within each chapter of this book, and the way that they relate to each other within a system, we liken this to a tree (see Figure 14.1).

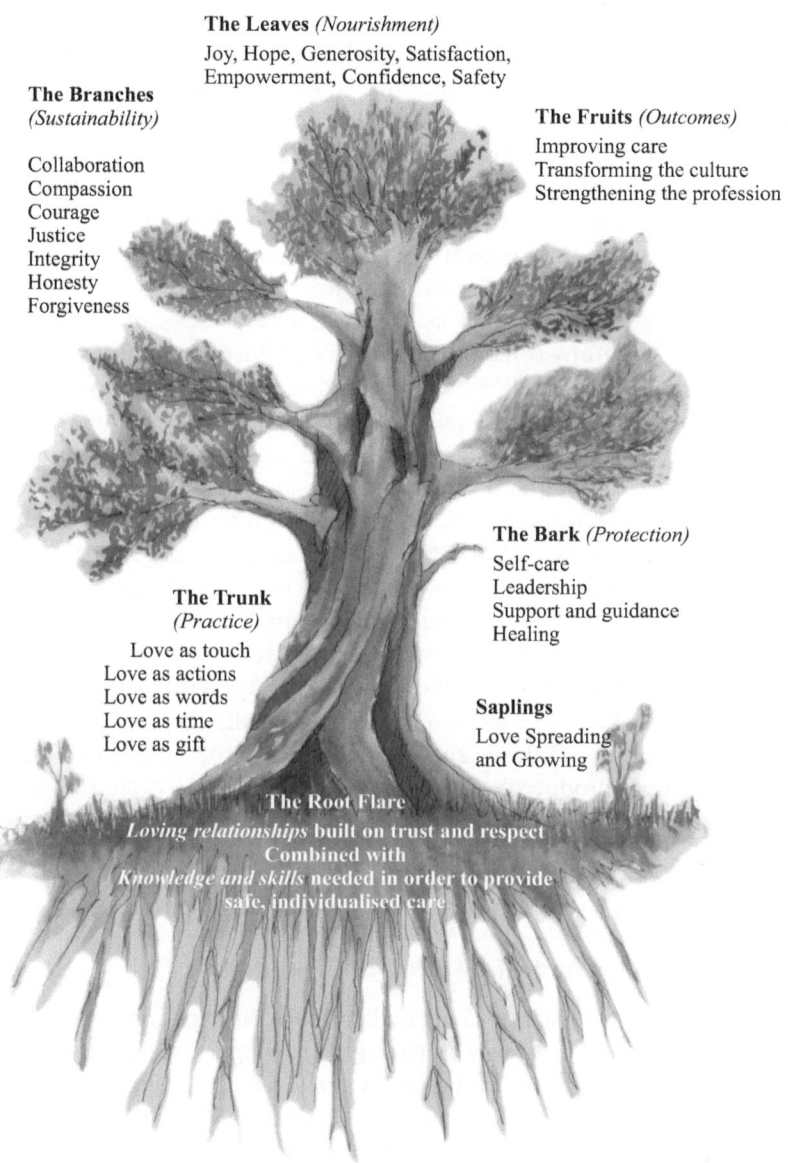

The Leaves *(Nourishment)*
Joy, Hope, Generosity, Satisfaction,
Empowerment, Confidence, Safety

The Branches
(Sustainability)

Collaboration
Compassion
Courage
Justice
Integrity
Honesty
Forgiveness

The Fruits *(Outcomes)*
Improving care
Transforming the culture
Strengthening the profession

The Bark *(Protection)*
Self-care
Leadership
Support and guidance
Healing

The Trunk
(Practice)
Love as touch
Love as actions
Love as words
Love as time
Love as gift

Saplings
Love Spreading
and Growing

The Root Flare
Loving relationships built on trust and respect
Combined with
Knowledge and skills needed in order to provide
safe, individualised care

The Roots *(Love as)*
Caring, Energy, Value, Meaning, Choice

FIGURE 14.1   Tree of love in midwifery

The roots of the tree go deep, and they represent the love that drives or guides us as explored in Part I of this book: love as caring; as energy; as a value or principle; as meaning and as a choice. The part of the tree where the roots join to the trunk is called the root flare. This represents the fundamentals of midwifery: knowledge, skills, and the ability to develop trusting relationships. Without these, we are not midwives at all, and this is why midwifery education and a loving approach within midwifery education, are absolutely key to love in midwifery. The trunk represents midwifery practice, and it reflects Part II of this book in that it incorporates touch, actions, words (communication), time, and gift as the manifestations of loving practice. The bark of the tree represents the protection we need as midwives. On a tree the bark is an insulator and a barrier to damage and physical threats. If it is damaged, then the tree becomes stressed and vulnerable to disease. But bark wounds can heal if they are not too severe. Like a tree many of us have had some knocks and carry the gnarly knots and scars left by some of the things we have encountered along the way. As midwives we also need protection, and in Part III, we explored how this comes from self-care (love of self); love from our colleagues and from professional and organisational support, guidance, and leadership. Without this we lose the ability to heal, and we may not be able to protect ourselves against stress, disease, and trauma. The branches symbolise the sustainability of our practice, grounded in collaboration, compassion, courage, justice, integrity, honesty, and forgiveness. The leaves of a tree harness light to provide nourishment and on our tree they represent what nourishes us as individuals and as a profession; they represent the sustenance we draw from joy, hope, generosity, satisfaction, empowerment, confidence, and safety. With respect to midwifery, the fruits of our love are continuously improving all aspects of care, transforming the maternity culture and strengthening the midwifery profession. Ultimately, trees produce fruits that sow seed in order to reproduce themselves and create new saplings. Therefore, fruit represents long term growth and renewal. In our tree of love we see this as the spreading and growing of love in midwifery.

Transformation of midwifery through Love

Ultimately, love enhances the care and enriches the experiences of those in our care as well as our experience of caring, nurturing a sense of community and support among colleagues and teams. Love is readily available to us because it is inside us and not something out there that we need to find. One of the most compelling reasons to practise midwifery lovingly is that it feels good. Providing care that comes from a place of love is pleasurable. It is not just the receiver of care that benefits; it is heart-warming, satisfying, and fulfilling for the care provider. Loving midwifery care is good for midwives.

Love is inherently human, and most people believe that, when all is said and done, love is the thing that matters most in life. Love can guide us as humans but sometimes it is overshadowed by the demands made of us as professionals and employees. These demands are important and cannot be ignored but to forget our humanness is perilous. We argue that midwives need to be human beings first, professionals second, and employees third. Keeping our priorities in that order will benefit everybody. Unfortunately, investigations into failings in maternity care are littered with examples of midwives and other maternity care workers failing to do this. We can only humanise care if we keep our humanness at the forefront of what we do as professionals and employees.

In maternity services, we have tried learning from distress, disappointment, and disaster and the evidence is that it is not an effective way of problem solving or changing the culture in maternity services. It is time for a radical new approach. Now, more than ever before, it is time to embrace love as an active practice to guide us towards a more compassionate, just, and hopeful future. It is already happening; there are many role models out there taking their love into their work every day when they are caring for women and families, their colleagues, and themselves or when they are carrying out their roles in leadership, education, research, and policy. Now it needs to spread and grow. You will know that love is not always easy; it will be demanding and takes courage. It is not something to be achieved or ticked-off; as noted by Clare in Chapter 2, it is not perfection but progress. Yet it is always worthwhile because the benefits are so great. It will take time, but midwife-by-midwife, team-by-team, service-by-service we believe that love is the catalyst for a much-needed transformation in midwifery and maternity services.

References

Byrom, S., & Downe, S. (2010). "She sort of shines": midwives' accounts of "good" midwifery and "good" leadership. *Midwifery*, *26*(1), 126–137. https://doi.org/10.1016/j.midw.2008.01.011

Goldman, J., & Wong, B. M. (2020). Nothing soft about 'soft skills': core competencies in quality improvement and patient safety education and practice. *BMJ Quality and Safety*, *29*(8), 619–622. https://doi.org/10.1136/bmjqs-2019-010512

Kuipers, Y, Greig, Y, & Norris, G. (2025). Human communication elements of the continuity of midwife care newsletter: A descriptive case report. *Creative Nursing*, *31*(1). https://doi.org/10.1177/10784535241298275

Parlamis, J., & Monnot, M. J. (2019). Getting to the CORE: Putting an end to the term "Soft Skills". *Journal of Management Inquiry*, *28*(2), 225–227. https://doi.org/10.1177/1056492618818023

Point of Care Foundation. (2024). *The point of care announces humanising care fellowships*. https://www.pointofcarefoundation.org.uk/news/the-point-of-care-foundation-announces-humanising-care-fellowships/#:~:text=outcomes%20for%20everyone.%E2%80%9D-,Juliet%20Rayment,as%20a%20freelance%20research%20consultant

Raham Project. (2024). *Helping ethnic minority families*. https://rahamproject.org.uk/

INDEX

Pages in *italics* refer to figures and pages in **bold** refer to tables.